# FACING THE FIRE

PAT HARDISON

ROSE
& PEARL
Publishing

Facing the Fire

Copyright © 2025 Rose & Pearl Publishing, LLC. All rights reserved.

No part of this publication may be reproduced, stored in a retrieval system, or transmitted in any form or by any means—electronic, mechanical, photocopy, recording, or otherwise—without prior written permission of the publisher, except in the case of brief quotations embodied in critical articles or reviews.

Trade Paperback ISBN: 979-8-9894343-6-7

Hardcover ISBN: 979-8-9894343-8-1

eBook ISBN: 979-8-9894343-7-4

Audiobook ISBN: 979-8-9894343-9-8

Scripture quotations are from The ESV® Bible (The Holy Bible, English Standard Version®), © 2001 by Crossway, a publishing ministry of Good News Publishers. Used by permission. All rights reserved.

Cover art/design: Kevin Pitts

Back-matter photograph: © Brandee Lott Photography. Used by permission.

Editing: Gregory Gobin

Interior design/typesetting: Rose & Pearl Publishing

Publisher: Rose & Pearl Publishing, LLC • Senatobia, MS • roseandpearlpublishing.com

Permissions & inquiries: support@roseandpearl.net

First edition, September 2025

Printed in the United States of America

10 9 8 7 6 5 4 3 2 1

This is a work of nonfiction. Some names and identifying details have been changed to protect privacy. Events are recounted from the author's memory, contemporaneous notes, and interviews.

The views and opinions expressed in this book are those of the author and do not necessarily reflect the views of the publisher.

This book describes the author's personal medical experiences and opinions. It is not intended as medical advice. Consult a qualified professional for guidance regarding any medical condition.

*To those in danger of losing hope—
and to all who face the fire.*

# CONTENTS

| | |
|---|---|
| Prologue | 1 |
| PART I<br>Into the Fire | 3 |
| PART II<br>The Man I Was | 25 |
| PART III<br>The Mirror | 65 |
| PART IV<br>My Undoing | 71 |
| PART V<br>The Mirror Breaks | 127 |
| PART VI<br>The Man I Became | 135 |
| PART VII<br>The Cost of Surviving | 179 |
| Epilogue | 194 |
| Photos | 197 |
| Timeline of Events | 199 |
| *Acknowledgments* | 203 |
| *About the Author* | 207 |
| *Publisher's Note* | 209 |

*I will refine them as one refines silver,*
*and test them as gold is tested.*
*They will call upon my name, and I will answer them.*

**- Zechariah 13:9 (ESV)**

# PROLOGUE

They say that your life flashes before your eyes when you are facing death. All I saw was melting shingles.

By the time we got there, the house was already engulfed in flames. But what do you do when you are faced with a distraught husband screaming that his wife is still inside? I looked at Matt.

"Let's go."

We pulled on our air packs and headed into the fire. As we walked through the bedroom at the far side of the house, we saw no one inside. Before we could make it out of the room and into the kitchen, heat exploded from overhead. In the chaos, I reached for my partner, my hand brushing against his sleeve before the weight of the collapsing roof knocked it away. Heat seared through my gear. I'm not sure how I got back to the window—but frantic arms yanked me through it. I landed hard. People rushed forward, trying to put out the fire consuming my head and shoulders.

Chaos turned to pandemonium. I could hear their shouts. "Help's coming man, hang in there. Pat, Pat, can you hear me? Talk to me, man.

I gasped for breath, trying to pull oxygen into my lungs, but it seemed hopeless. I didn't realize how precious oxygen was until my supply seemed to decrease drastically. It would have been wiser to reserve my breath, but I didn't care. I grabbed Bricky Cole and pulled him close. "Take care of Chrissi and the kids. Promise me."

"I will, man, I will. But hang with me. Don't give up on me right now, man. Help's coming, the chopper is on the way. Talk to me, Pat. You have to keep talking to stay awake, okay? Do it for Chrissi and the kids."

And for a split second, I thought, *This is it. This is the end.*

But little did I know, what I thought was the end, was really the beginning in disguise.

# PART I
## INTO THE FIRE

# 1

## THAT'S NOT PAT

When I glanced up into the mirror, what I saw broke me. I didn't recognize the thing staring back. It wasn't a face. And in that moment, I understood Chrissi's words from that afternoon six months before. "That's not Pat. That can't be my husband!"

When doctors finally cut pinholes in the skin grafts covering my eyes, it was the first time I'd seen anything since the day of the fire. I was at my house, not paying attention, and walked in front of a mirror and looked up.

No ears. No lips. No nose. No eyebrows or eyelids or hair. Just shiny, puckered skin. Like melted wax pulled from a campfire. I did not know how bad everything was until that moment. Not the weeks in the burn unit, not the doctors' words that offered little hope, not the torturous skin grafts. It was what I saw in the mirror that truly told me how deep the injuries actually went. *My God, Pat, what have you done to yourself?*

You don't realize how much of your identity lives in your face. In the tilt of your smile. The way your eyes squint when you laugh. The nose that makes you look like your dad. The jawline that reminds him of your grandpa.

Until it is gone.

And it was all gone, lost in the smoke and flames of that fire on Wheeler Road. Yet, it was just the beginning of all I had to lose, and the decades-long fight to try and get it back.

---

CHRISSI HAD BEEN on the phone with her aunt, chatting to pass the time while she cleaned the house. She had been in "the hunting room," a study where I kept all my hunting gear, decorated with a camouflage couch and trophy animals. I had my desk and computer in there as well, and it was where I would sit and pay our bills each month. She was vacuuming while our kids played around her feet. She didn't want to get off the phone with her aunt to answer when Travis McDonald, my friend who worked with me at the tire store, began calling. But after multiple missed calls, she decided to check if something was wrong, just in case.

"Hey, Travis, what's up?"

"Do you know where Pat is?"

"He should be back at the store with you by now. He stopped back by here after lunch, and said he was heading that way. Has he not made it back yet?" Her chest became tight with concern.

"He did make it back, yes, but someone called and told me that he had been hurt. He was called out on a fire right after he got here. They said he had been flown out to The Med."

"That's ridiculous. Someone would have called me if that was true. I'll call Pat and find out what is going on." But her calls to my phone went unanswered. That wasn't uncommon though, as I wouldn't have answered if I were still on scene or even back at the firehouse. Maybe they got the people mixed up, details confused in the chaos of a fire and the resulting phone tag to spread the news. It can't be Pat who is hurt. She began calling Chief Copeland, but he wasn't answering either. Desperate, she just kept calling, over and over, until finally he picked up. "It's okay, Chrissi. We have sent someone to get your mom from work. Your family will be at your house soon. Then, you can go..."

She threw the phone to the ground and ran outside to the garage apartment where my brother Shannon was living. As her knees trembled, the words tumbled out, letting him know why a mass of friends and family were pulling into our driveway. The small-town grapevine spread the news of the tragedy quicker than lightning.

No, they hadn't called her. They didn't want her to be alone with the kids when she found out that I had sustained injuries so severe that I had to be flown to our regional trauma center in Memphis, known to locals as "The Med."

THE ROAR of rotor blades filled the sky. Medics had dropped to their knees beside me, strapping me to a board, lifting me up and loading me into the chopper. I felt like I was floating—somewhere between pain and nothing.

A woman's voice broke through the noise.

"My name is Paula. What's your name?"

"Pat." My voice was rough and hoarse. She was leaning over me, starting IVs and who knows what else.

"Pat, are you married? Do you have kids?"

I nodded, but my voice cracked.

"Stay with me. Tell me their names."

"Alison."

"Alison! That's great. How old is she?"

"Six."

"You have more?"

"Dalton…" A coughing fit interrupted me. "…and Averi."

"You're doing great, Pat. I need to you stay awake, okay? How old are they?"

"Four…and…two."

Then I heard the pilot.

"How's he doing?"

"Talking. Sort of. Hard to say. Not sure if he knows what he is saying."

Anger flared in my chest. Weak as I was, I still had my mind.

"I know how old my kids are," I rasped.

"Of course you do, Pat," Paula whispered.

But I didn't want to talk about them anymore. I couldn't. Thinking about them, about what they'd do without me, was worse than the pain. I didn't want to imagine their birthdays without me there. The empty chair at Christmas. Chrissi tryin' to hold it all together.

*Ask me about anything else*, I thought. *Just not them.*

SHANNON DROVE Chrissi and my parents forty-one miles to the hospital. "Can't you drive any faster?" She begged. Her panicked voice shook.

"No need to speed and get us all killed. Better to get there in one piece."

But she wanted to scream at him, reach over with her foot and press the accelerator all the way to the floorboard. Every second she had to wait to find out what was happening was like torture. Instead, she sat frozen in fear, praying that her worst nightmares weren't about to come true, that she would not be left alone to raise our kids, who were at home with her sister. She had no idea that the reality would be worse than she could have even imagined.

RIGHT BEFORE I landed at The Med, the flight nurse leaned in close and said, "Now when we touch down, there's gonna be an entire team waiting. They're gonna do a lot of things real fast. Just be ready."

I didn't know what else to expect. The flight nurse had already started IVs, pain meds, and tried to intubate me. I had warned her, "You can't do that…I'll throw up…ain't much room…" She opted to let the hospital arrival team deal with whatever might come up out of my stomach.

Sure enough, soon as we landed and they flung open that chopper door, I saw this big guy standing there, silhouetted against the light, holding a tube. Didn't say a word. Just leaned in and jammed that thing straight down my throat.

And just like I warned her—I threw up. Everywhere.

That was the last thing I remember saying for a long time. After that, the talking stopped.

THE CHAPLAIN MET Chrissi and our parents at the emergency room door. He led them to a small chapel and asked if he could pray with them, but Chrissi couldn't even bow her head. She just stood there, frozen, waiting for somebody to tell her if I was even alive. How bad must it be if a chaplain meets the family at the door and begins praying with them?

"Please just tell me if he is alive?" Chrissi begged the chaplain.

"They have him in the back and are working on him. He was alive before I came to meet you, but they are not expecting him to make it. I am so sorry."

She knew it wasn't going to be good news, but she had hoped for smoke inhalation, some burns on arms or back, but not this. This was a nightmare. Maybe she could wake herself up.

"Can I see him...you know...before..." She couldn't bring herself to finish the sentence.

"I really don't think that is a good idea. The burns are extensive, and you don't want that to be the last image you have of your husband."

"If he is alive, I want to see him! To tell him I love him one last time. Please!"

"Let me see what I can do." The chaplain left, taking all the hope in the room with him.

THE DOCTORS finally agreed to let her see me, for what might be one last time. Orderlies led her down a long, bright hallway. Nobody else around except our parents.

When the double doors opened, they wheeled out a stretcher with me lying there, able to hear her, but not communicate.

'That's not Pat!" Chrissi exclaimed, her eyes wide, as she stared down at the stretcher. "That can't be my husband! It looks more like someone put a Boston butt on the grill and left it too long." She took a shaky breath trying to take in the sight before her. A body, covered in a sheet, with a lump of meat where the head should be, smoking and oozing. Her voice was barely above a whisper, "What is that dripping off the stretcher?"

The doctor spoke slowly, keeping his voice calm as he replied, "I assure you, this is Pat. And what you see oozing down the stretcher is his skin melting. With burns as severe as these, your body continues to burn for a few weeks after the initial injury."

I had full-thickness burns over my entire head and most of my shoulders, which means that the burn went all the way through all layers of skin, not just the surface. That burns all the nerve endings as well, so I couldn't initially feel the pain. I had burned part of my airway, and that is usually what kills you. But they were able to keep my airway open. They could not put bandages on me at first, as there was too much swelling. What we kept hearing, repeatedly from every doctor and specialist, was that most people cannot survive an accident like this. Yet here I was, surviving.

The doctor reached out and put his hand on my wife's shoulder. "We did warn you seeing him might not be a good idea, but we didn't want to deny you that request. Let's get you and your parents somewhere quiet. I know this is a lot to process."

THEY LED them back to a waiting room. In shock, Chrissi went into autopilot, functioning like everything was fine, shutting away the part of herself that wanted to crumble into a ball and come apart at the seams. She kept visiting, talking to people. Hospital staff moved the family upstairs to a conference room because so many people began arriving. Hundreds of friends, fellow firefighters, and other first responders who had heard and wanted to show their support.

News crews kept calling. And she kept talking, and moving, even laughing as if she were in a dream and not a nightmare. Said it felt like she was walking around inside a movie of someone else's life, playing a part with no connection to reality. She shared with the media what she knew, which at that point wasn't much, and just kept going. Wondering what on earth had happened in those few hours we had been apart?

# 2

## THE FIRE

It had been just a regular Wednesday. I swung by the fire station early that morning, as was my routine, to grab a cup of coffee and catch up with the guys. The place smelled of diesel and burnt toast—comforting in a strange way. The old coffee pot hissed and sputtered, spitting out a dark, bitter brew we all drank like it was gold. We talked shop, shared a few laughs, and then I headed out, planning to open up the store.

As I was driving to the store, I heard a voice, clear as day. "Today, things are going to change." I thought it was strange, but I struggled off the uneasy feeling I had in my stomach. Maybe I imagined it, I told myself. Looking back, I see how God was giving me a warning, or maybe even a choice. Do what I had always done, and my life would change forever, or I could heed this divine warning, and maybe not travel down the dark road ahead of me. I ignored the voice. I never was good at listening to what others told me to do.

AROUND LUNCHTIME, I drove over to Coleman's Bar-B-Que, where the smoke hung heavy in the air and the smell of hickory and pork hit you before you even got outta the truck. I ordered the usual—pulled pork plate with baked beans and slaw—and took a seat with a few of the local boys. The place buzzed with chatter, folks from nearby shops and businesses squeezing in their break before the afternoon rush. Forks scraped plates, tea glasses clinked, and the waitress hollered out orders like she owned the joint.

After I wiped the last bit of sauce off my mouth with a paper napkin, I got back in the truck and swung by the fire station one more time. Just check in. Just say hey. I figured the rest of the day would be spent back at the shop, selling tires and chatting with customers like always.

As I left that second time, I called over my shoulder, "Y'all need to find us a good fire today."

Just a joke.

I wish I'd never said it.

I HADN'T BEEN BACK at the tire store long when the two-tone alarm sounded on my pager. That shrill, heart-pounding buzz lit me up like electricity. I jumped up, bolted through the office door, and tore down Main Street in my truck, weaving through traffic like a man late to his own wedding.

With an almost all-volunteer force, how fast you got to the station mattered. First ones there rode the truck. First ones there fought the fire. The rest just stood by, waiting, listening, aching for the stories they'd hear later. I didn't want to hear about it. I wanted to *be* there.

Chief Copeland was already at the bay doors when I skidded into the lot. Other firefighters arrived from every direction, peeling out of work shirts and pulling on gear. Chief didn't waste time.

"Hot one out on Wheeler Road," he barked. "Hernando's already on two house fires and this is their third. We've got to go help."

Wheeler Road was in the small town of Love, just a dot on the map across the county line where trees outnumbered mailboxes. We drove through it regularly up Highway 51 on the way to the larger cities like Hernando, Southaven, and Memphis. We never crossed the county line for a call unless it was an emergency. But I knew when Chief's voice dropped like that, it was serious.

Matt Hale, Jason McAbee, Bricky Cole, Clay Moore, and I climbed into the truck with Chief. We paired up based on where we sat. Usually, you ended up with whoever landed next to you. Brother Clay, as we called him, had been up front, but slid into the back before we rolled out. That change put me next to Matt. The youngest of our crew, Matt had joined the squad when he was 18, about three years before. Guy had just become old enough to drink legally, and there he was heading out on a serious house fire that wasn't even his first.

RULE NUMBER ONE IN FIREFIGHTING: Whatever the dispatcher says, it probably ain't what you'll find. People call in panicked. Can't remember which side of the house is on fire. Don't know where their kids are. Forget about gas lines, dogs, locked doors. You show up and start from scratch.

We pulled up to the scene, an old mobile home with additions wrapped around it like a patchwork quilt, that kind of construction that makes fires burn hotter and collapse quicker. Flames were already licking through the roof on the east side, roaring like a freight train. Smoke curled into the gray sky, thick and angry.

Matt and I grabbed a line and went in through the front and made an initial sweep of the house, finding no one inside. When we came out, a man was jumping up and down outside, wild-eyed, shouting that his wife was still inside. Two cars sat in the gravel drive. That checked out. But it had taken nearly thirty minutes from tone to arrival. First we had to get to the station, then haul it eleven miles up Highway 51 to Wheeler Road. If she *was* inside... was it even possible she was still alive? How did we miss her on the initial sweep? I made the call for Matt and I to go back in. I knew I wouldn't be able to live with myself if she had been in there and we had missed her on the initial sweep. We grabbed our air packs and began looking for a way in.

. . .

AIR PACKS CAME ALONG in the '70s and '80s, but the old Memphis firemen will tell you they had them on the truck but weren't allowed to use them. Back then, firemen never wore air packs. That may be why so many of them later died from lung cancer, from all the carcinogens they breathed in over years on the job.

Then came the Nomex hood. Picture a ski mask worn under your air mask and helmet. It's thin, but it gives you just enough protection, and just enough warning. If you start feeling heat on your ears through it, that's your signal: Time to get the hell out. That's how you judge the temperature in a room. If your ears start burning, you're probably pushing a thousand degrees in there.

Some guys wear two hoods, thinking it'll protect them better, but that just dulls that little warning system. That's the kind of thing you learn over time, from experience. That's why older firemen are supposed to teach the new ones, pass down the knowledge that keeps you alive.

Back then, we didn't have thermal imaging cameras or helmet-mounted HUDs, those cameras that can tell you exactly where someone is inside. Nowadays, if someone is lying on the floor, that camera will pick them up. You don't have to crawl around blindly searching in a blackout. Now you have one eye on a screen mounted to your helmet, letting you see as you move. Then we had no infrared readouts or fancy gadgets. Just our eyes, our instincts, and each other.

It wasn't likely someone could have been inside without gear and still be alive, but I was determined to look anyway.

WE TRIED the front door first, but the fire on the east side was like a wall we couldn't get through. Matt and I peeled off to the west, looking for another way in. Found a bedroom window. I smashed the glass, cleared the shards, and climbed through, Matt right behind me. We pulled a line through with us and started sweeping. The smoke inside was thick, black, and choking, like soup. My mask filtered most of it, but every breath still burned like whiskey down the wrong pipe.

Most of the time in a fire, you can't see your hand in front of your face. That's why your partner stays close, touching your boot or trailing your hose. You move slow. Tap with your ax. Feel for bodies, doorframes, furniture. If your partner hits something, they break off, check it quick, then return.

We moved around the foot of the bed toward the hall door. My ears were burning through my Nomex hood. Time to get out.

We hadn't found anyone yet.

Then—*crack*.

The ceiling groaned. I looked up.

It came down in an instant. Burning rafters. Melting shingles. Ceiling tiles turned to shrapnel.

Something slammed into the back of my helmet. The blow knocked it clean off. I tried to call out, but smoke poured into my mouth, thick and bitter. I reached for Matt, but a beam knocked my arm away. He vanished in the black. I hit the floor hard, back near the bed.

Brother Clay and Jason were working the front of the house with a hose. They didn't know we'd come in from the side. Now we were getting pounded from both ends, water blasting in from the front, steam pushing down from the collapse.

That house had two roofs, one over the original trailer and another added during renovations. Fire trapped between them acted like a furnace, cooking the space until it gave way. That second roof fell like a trapdoor slamming shut.

I DON'T KNOW if I blacked out. Maybe I did. Everything was muffled, warped. Like being underwater. My helmet was gone. My gear was burning. I could smell leather, plastic, flesh. Me—*burning*. A sweet, sickening scent I'll never forget.

I tried to push the ceiling off me. My ears screamed. I crawled toward the window, instinct taking over. No thoughts. Just motion. I had to get out. Wherever Matt was, I couldn't tell; we were on our own.

Then hands—*real hands*—grabbed me, pulled me through. Air hit my face like ice. I collapsed outside, gasping, the sun blinding me.

Voices shouted. Gear thudded. Someone screamed my name. Water hit me, putting out the fire.

I was sprawled in the grass, barely breathing, smoke rising off my back. Chief had already called in the chopper. "Firefighter down." The words rang out like a bell over the radio, setting everything in motion.

Bricky knelt beside me. I grabbed his coat. My voice was barely a whisper.

"Take care of Chrissi and the kids. Promise me."

"I will, man. I will. Just hang on. Stay with me. Help's coming."

"THE DOCTOR'S HERE," Chrissi whispered, nodding towards the double doors of the hospital conference room. People parted as the man in the white coat headed towards my family.

"He's still hanging in there. We will need to transfer him to the burn unit, but there aren't any beds there now. We will get him there as soon as we can. You need to know, the next 48 hours are critical. We will begin treating the burns the best we can and see what we are working with, but we still don't know if he will make it, so I want you to begin preparing yourself in case. We have the Chaplin and social workers here to help you with anything you or your family need."

"Can I see him again?"

"Sure, I can take you to him."

The doctor walked Chrissi back to the ER. One of the nurses met her and let her see me again, if only for a few minutes.

"We are about to debride the skin, so let me walk you back to the waiting room," the nurse finally told Chrissi, stepping towards the curtain, indicating for Chrissi to follow.

"What does that mean—'debride the skin'?"

"We scrub down to where the burn stops."

Chrissi's nose crinkled, "That sounds awful, and painful."

"He is on Dilaudid and morphine, which will make him as comfortable as possible, but it will still hurt, yes."

"I'm going to stay. I want to be here as long as I can."

The nurse looked at her and gave a sad smile. "You can't be in here while we perform the procedure, so it's best if you head back to the waiting room.

"I need to be with him," Chrissi insisted. But the nurse told her absolutely not, so she stood outside the room, as close as she was allowed to be.

When they started, I screamed until I passed out, the pain excruciating despite the heavy medication. Chrissi had to leave. The screams were just too much. Would have been too much for anyone.

LATER THAT NIGHT, when the crowd that had been there most of evening had finally drifted away back to their homes, Chrissi broke down. Said she just melted down in a puddle of tears right in the middle of a conversation with our parents. Couldn't hold it in anymore. They found a nurse and got her something to help calm her down, and after that, she got quiet. Numb.

She told me later that it felt like she lived in a fog for years after that. Said there's a point where your brain just refuses to take in anymore. So, you float. You smile. You nod. But you're not really there.

Nurses settled Chrissi and our parents in the intensive care waiting room, which had recliners that laid back so you could try to get some sleep between visiting hours. Chrissi couldn't stand being away from our kids for the night, wanting to hold and comfort them, but she didn't want to scare them with her tears or worries either. And neither she nor our parents could stand to be away from the hospital, not knowing what the next minute or hour might hold.

. . .

So much of what happened that day is a blur. In a fire, everything is confusion. Smoke blinds you and clouds your vision. Turnouts are bulky and designed for heat resistance and protection, not ease of movement. Adrenaline and training flood your system causing you to react from instinct, only able to diagnose later what external factor caused you to respond.

This was also before 9-11.

Before the outpouring of love and money provided more advanced equipment and training to strapped firehouses in small towns.

Before our fire department would replace volunteers with professionals who were trained in more advanced ways to evaluate the balance of risk versus reward in saving life and property.

Also...it was before I would learn what it truly meant to suffer.

# 3

# THE WORLD COLLAPSES

I remained parked in a drug-induced haze in the ER while my family hung around in the various waiting areas of the hospital. My burns were confined mostly to my head and upper shoulders. From the chest down, I was fine. Friends came and went, delivering food and fresh clothes to my family, and updates on the kids back home. Yet, I wasn't allowed to see most of the visitors. Didn't know most of them were there at first. I did not have bandages covering any of my burns. This was to allow the swelling to go down. Thus, from the chest up, I was just one large open wound, putting me at a higher risk for infection. Everyone had to be gowned and gloved just to come in.

I'd never felt so alone. Couldn't see. Couldn't move because of all the tubes. Couldn't have many visitors. Couldn't really talk to them if they came in. But the whole time, I *could hear everything*. My ears were gone—burned off in the fire like my nose and eyelids. But the mechanics inside my ears still worked. The nurses would leave the TV on for me as my only company. The reports of crime and bad weather became the background noise to the pain in my body and heart.

I lay there, day after day, trapped in the inferno of my own body, listening to machines beep and nurses whisper. Sometimes I'd hear folks crying outside my room and wonder if they knew something I didn't. I wasn't scared, not exactly. It felt like I'd already died, and my body hadn't caught up yet.

I wish I could say I was praying. That I felt some kind of peace, like God was sitting there in that hospital room with me. But the truth? I wasn't thinking about God. I was thinking about how everything hurt, and how I wanted out of that hospital, in a car or a hearse — I didn't much care which. I didn't ask *Why me?* I asked *Why now? Why like this?* I'd been the one running in to help. I had young kids I still needed to raise and a company to run. And now I couldn't even see my own hands or speak my kids' names out loud. If God was there, I couldn't feel Him. Not then. He had tried to warn me, and I hadn't listened. Yet, He had saved me from death. But for what? To live the rest of my life like this—a deformed vegetable?

When I was awake, I was tortured with pain and thoughts of 'what if?' And when the medicine lulled me into a fitful sleep, I was tortured with nightmares of the fire and people dying because of my choices. I didn't have a concept of what the future would hold, or even if there would be a future. The present was filled only with pain. So, my mind would drift to the past. Should I have gone into the house? Why did I go in when I knew it was not possible for someone still to be alive inside? Did they ever find her? Did Matt get out? Was he hurt like I was—or worse, gone? What could I have done differently? What went wrong?

SIX DAYS after I arrived at The Med, I listened as early morning news shows shared breaking coverage with the world that at 8:46 a.m. EST a plane hit the north tower of the World Trade Center. Then another one hit the South Tower. Then one hit the Pentagon. One went down in a field in Pennsylvania. I heard the reports, the news of the firefighters running into the buildings to save those trapped inside and never coming out. Jimmie Neal, one of my best friends and among the few allowed in the room with me, insisted that I cut the TV off, that I didn't need to hear the reports of the dead firefighters. I couldn't change the channel and avoid the news. It was on all of them. Not having the TV on was the only option. I couldn't argue with him about it, tell him I wanted to know what was happening, feel connected to the outside world, even if it was literally falling down around people just like that house had fallen down around me. All I could do was scribble on a notepad or dry-erase board, hoping that the letters I could not see formed the words I wanted to say, cry, scream.

ONE OF THE only people who understood my desperate need to hear what was happening as the world as we knew it changed in an instant was my sister, Lori. She was living in Jacksonville, Florida, when my world collapsed. Her husband, Clark, was a Navy fighter pilot, deployed somewhere near the Horn of Africa. Chrissi had called her as people had been arriving at our house, panicked, screaming into the phone, trying to explain what was happening with no answers to give. I was burned. Bad. Didn't know if I was alive or dead. Lori said they both ended up crying into the phone, miles apart, scared out of their minds.

Lori called her community officer's wife to pass word along to Clark about the accident. There was no easy way to reach somebody out at sea, not back then. All she had were emails and twenty-minute calls once a month if you were lucky. But her friend's husband had a phone in his stateroom. He found Clark and let him and Lori talk. They both just cried and prayed.

By then it had been too late in the day for Lori to drive. Twelve hours from Florida to Memphis with two little girls wasn't safe, especially not in Lori's emotional state. She called her in-laws and said she'd be on the road at daylight. But they stepped in and bought her plane tickets instead. Three of them. Said she needed to be there fast, not exhausted.

The next morning, one of her friends drove Lori and the girls to the airport. She flew into Memphis where her mother-in-law picked them up and took them straight to The Med. For the next several days, she stayed with her in-laws while she visited the hospital each day to care for our parents and Chrissi.

When Lori came to visit me the day of the attacks, I scribbled on the pad next to me, "Where's Clark?" I imagined they were already being given orders to move towards this terrorist threat.

"I'm not sure. They were somewhere near the Horn of Africa when I told him about the accident. I am sure they are moving back into the Gulf."

I began writing on the dry-erase board. "Tell...him..." What little strength I had faded, and my hand was getting weaker.

"Tell him what, Pat?"

*Finish what you started, Pat.* So, I did. "...to kick ass," I wrote.

"Get better, and tell him yourself." I heard her chuckle weakly.

I didn't know how she was doing it. There she was, holding it together while her brother was fighting between life and death, and now, her husband was heading into a war zone. My sister was fighting to keep her world from collapsing as well.

I also needed to know that Matt's world hadn't come crashing down. Actually, that was the first question I had when I could communicate. Had he made it out? Was he alive? I was the one who made the call to go back in, and as Captain, he was under my command. I always protected my guys, so I felt responsible. I wasn't sure I was going to be able to live with myself if he hadn't made it out, or if he was hurt like I was. I scribbled what I hoped was "Matt?" on the dry-erase board and held my breath for the response.

"He's fine," my friend Zander told me. "Got out right behind you. Came running around from the back of the house, yelling that you were still inside. But they'd already pulled you out. Said he tried to find you, but a gap opened up in the smoke and flames, and he knew he had to take it."

Thank God! The weight of not knowing had already settled deep. I was so grateful I would never have to find out how I would have responded had the news been different.

And the lady? The one we went in after? Turned out she wasn't even home. She'd gone walking down the road to fish without leaving a note for her husband. He had assumed she was inside, but she walked up later like nothing had happened, asking what all the fuss was about. I mean, I was glad she was alive, of course. But I'd be lying if I said it didn't hit me hard. If I'd known she wasn't in there, I never would've made the call to go inside. But what-ifs don't heal burns. They just settle in your chest and make it ache.

AND FOR THE next two weeks, as my body continued to burn from the inside out, we waited. In that hospital, and across the country. We waited.

To get treatment.
To get answers.
To be moved to the burn unit.
To see if there were still survivors.
To have surgeries.
To find out America's response.
...To wake up from this nightmare.

# PART II
# THE MAN I WAS

# 4

# THE FIREFIGHTER

While the firefighters in New York City were making front-page news around the world, firefighters that I had served with, and many that I had never met, were coming by the hospital to show me their support. Some were allowed to scrub up and come in, but most would just check on Chrissi and send their best wishes. Although I appreciated the company, sometimes I felt crowded. Maybe it was the unknown of what was ahead. Or maybe it was being confined to a bed that felt suffocating. And the hourly checks of my vital signs didn't help.

The nurse wrestled with putting the blood pressure cuff around my arm as Jimmie moved out of her way but then went to my other side. I felt sandwiched. Between him breathing heavy while hovering over me, and the sound of Velcro ripping again so she could try another spot on my arm, I was desperate for someone to talk. Finally, Jimmie spoke. "Ronnie Warren stopped by this morning," he said. I thought about reaching for the dry-erase board but didn't have the energy to write. "He's taking it hard."

SIX YEARS BEFORE, on a Sunday morning at church, he had stopped me in the foyer with a smile on his face and a question that changed everything.

"Would you like to become a firefighter?" he asked.

I had Ronnie for shop class in high school and gave him a hard time. He was a good teacher and apparently, very forgiving. Giving me an opportunity like that showed that he didn't hold any of my antics against me.

"Never really thought about it," I told him. "But it might be alright."

THE SENATOBIA FIRE DEPARTMENT needed recruits, and he had figured I'd be good for the job. I had been only twenty, newly married to my first wife Rebecca, and we were expecting a child. Rebecca's granddad and uncles were firefighters, so I'd heard about firefighting plenty at family get-togethers. They'd swap stories about engine trouble and car wrecks and house blazes, and I'd nod along but never really saw it as my world. Still, I was curious. My buddy Neal Copeland and I decided to join up together. Neal joining wasn't a big surprise. His dad was on the force. For Neal, it was in his blood. For me? I guess I just thought it would be cool to try, and maybe another place where I could hang out with my friends.

THE PROCESS WAS SIMPLE ENOUGH. We went down to the station, sat with a few of the guys, and they interviewed us. No fancy application, just a simple background check. After a few questions, some laughter, and a firm handshake, you were in. If they accepted you, which they almost always did considering they mostly recruited the young guys in town they already knew, then you headed down to the state capital, filled out your paperwork, and got your gear.

I could understand why Ronnie may have felt partially responsible, but what he didn't realize was that it was because of him, I gained an extended family. After getting accepted, I learned that truth quickly. I learned the firehouse was a brotherhood like nothing I'd ever known. It was loud and messy and full of dark humor. But it was real. We would sit around the firehouse, drink coffee, and listen to the guys talk about past calls. The kinds of stories that make your palms sweat. Most mornings, I'd swing by just to have a cup before heading to the tire store. Then, I'd come back at lunch for another cup and to check in with the guys. It truly became my second home, and I didn't even realize it was happening at the time.

Not only did my family grow, but so did my knowledge. Although I attended the training classes in my free time, most training happened on the job. The older guys took us under their wings and taught us the tricks of the trade. Their stories of wrecks and blazes they'd worked gave us more insight than any textbook could ever do. They didn't always say much, but when they did, you listened. If a man with smoke scars and melted gear told you to use a left-hand search pattern, you didn't argue. As a new recruit, you spend a major portion of your time just shutting your mouth and listening, knowing that one day you will have stories of your own to tell and wisdom to pass on to those under you.

RIGHT BEFORE HALLOWEEN, Rebecca and I went to the hospital to check on the baby, and they ended up keeping us there. That's when I received my first page. First fire call as an official firefighter and my wife was in labor with my very first child. I hadn't fought a fire yet, so I didn't know what I was missing. Honestly, I didn't even hear the page at first; I was focused on everything happening at the hospital.

Alison's birth hadn't been an easy one. That kind of moment pulls your whole world into one room. I ignored the pager, my attention on my wife and my new baby girl. And I didn't regret it. She came into the world screaming, pink-faced, tiny fists clenched like she already had something to fight for. I remembered what Dad once told me about his reaction to my older sister being born. "When I first saw her, I thought she was the ugliest thing I ever saw," he said. He'd never seen a newborn before, didn't realize how rough the trip through the birth canal could be. But 30 minutes later, when her head rounded out a little, he said, "Then she was the most beautiful thing I ever saw." I now understood exactly what he meant.

ONLY A DAY or two after returning home with our baby, my pager went off again. This time it was a serious wreck out in the county. That was the first time I saw a dead body. That kind of thing sticks with you. Haunts you. I'd never seen a body without life in it that wasn't prepared for burial. There's something different about the way a person looks when their soul is gone. Like a corn husk without the cob inside. You walk up to the scene thinking you're tough enough, then you see their shoes in the road and wonder if they were headed home. And who they were heading home to? I didn't talk about it. Not then. Maybe not for years. But I remembered.

My first house fire came soon after. An old shotgun house. Somebody left a space heater too close to something flammable, and up it went. Neal was with me on that one. We were both still green, still figuring out how to keep from roasting ourselves. I remember the smell of smoke sticking in my clothes for days. You'd think it'd be awful, but to me, it smelled like purpose.

One of the first fires I really remember was a few months later, in December. It was so cold the water lines froze solid, and our turnouts turned to ice. We were young and dumb. It was a big house fire, and if the guy on the hose wasn't careful, he'd send so much pressure down the line that it could lift you off the ground. We learned fast to coil it up and sit on it to keep the pressure steady. Numb fingers. Numb toes. Steam rising off your shoulders in the dark. That was life, and we loved it. There's a strange kind of joy in getting knocked flat and standing back up. It makes you feel alive.

WHAT I ONCE THOUGHT WOULD BE A COOL pastime became an addiction, and the high volume of calls just kept feeding that addiction. Despite being a small-town fire department, we had more calls than you'd think. The casinos had come to Tunica, a town one county over on the muddy waters of the Mississippi, 30 miles west of Senatobia. That meant people gambling all night and drinking free booze, then trying to drive back home on these two-lane back roads when they couldn't tell a yellow line from a white one. We'd get called when they flipped their cars into ditches and needed to be cut out. We learned fast that the job wasn't just about flames. It was about wreckage—twisted metal, soaked carpets, the sound of crying babies, and the eerie silence of someone not making it.

The more calls I responded to, the more I began to realize that this wasn't just a volunteer job. This was something much bigger. I wasn't just selling tires or checking pay stubs. I was running into danger to help people. This was something that gave me purpose. Hell, this was something that gave me an identity.

At 25, I was promoted to Captain, which wasn't a position just handed to anybody. Other firefighters had to vote yes for that to happen, which made it even more special. It meant that they trusted me and knew that I could handle the extra responsibilities. It also meant an increase in pay—from nothing to a whopping $15 a call! But I wasn't in it for the money; I was in it for the thrill of being able to help somebody.

Maybe Ronnie had seen more than just an able body who could help the town. On paper, I had everything back then. A wife, a lucrative business. A successful man like that doesn't need to be volunteering at a small-town fire station. On paper, I didn't need it. But my heart told a different story. Ronnie was the man who helped me find my calling and helped me find fulfillment. I would always be grateful that he saw more in me than a kid cutting up in his shop class.

Every spare second, I was at the station or training. I made every call I could while still working at the tire store. I was living two lives—business owner by day, firefighter at heart. Dad used to joke, "If Pat was in the middle of having sex and that beeper went off, he'd get up and go to the fire." Embarrassing as that is, I'm not 100% sure he was wrong.

Then there it was. A familiar sound. BEEP. BEEP. BEEP. Time to grab the gear and go. But I couldn't move. I was stuck. I heard the nurse moving near my bed. "Nothing to worry about, just pressed the wrong button," she said. I must have dozed off for a minute. "Well since you're up, now is a perfect time to take your blood pressure again." I couldn't wait to get out of this hospital and back to the life I loved at home—playing with my kids and fighting fires with my friends.

# 5

# THE SON

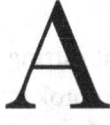s I lay there going in and out of a morphine-filled delirium, I could hear a deep voice in the room. "We'll figure this out, Pat. Just like we always do."
*Dad.*
Then there was a lady's voice that followed. "God, please give us all the strength to endure this battle that you lay before us."
*Mom.*
Ed and Elaine Hardison. I tried shifting to the voices but barely moved. "It's okay Pat, you just get your rest," my mom said. There was a feeling of sinking in place that overtook me. Imagine trying to stand up and something kept pushing you back down. I just gave up and lay there. They started talking to each other, and I wanted to jump in, but I couldn't. "What these doctor's need to do is figure out ASAP how to get him back home to Mississippi. The air there will do him good," he said. I didn't know if the Mississippi air held that power, but he was right about one thing. I missed home. Not just my house—my town. At this point, I wasn't sure if I was saved to serve a purpose or saved to suffer and then just die. Well, if I were going to die soon, I wouldn't want it to be in The Med. God, at least let my end be at the same place it all began. I faded deeper and before I knew it, there I was

back in my hometown. I could hear the church bells and almost feel the dirt from the roads sticking to the bottom of my boots, just like when I was a boy–back when I looked up to my dad. I mean, I appreciated him coming to see me now in the hospital, but my respect for him wasn't the same as when I was a little boy. Now he was a concerned dad supporting his burnt son in the hospital, but before... he was my hero.

ED GREW up a few miles west of Senatobia in the small community of Strayhorn, where there is neither a post office nor a stoplight. Where dirt roads and church bells set the rhythm of life. Around there, everybody knows everybody, and the church prayer list doubles as the grapevine. It's the kind of place where the local dentist moonlights as mayor, and summer nights are for Little League games coached by the school board superintendent.

Dad's father worked in heating and air until an accident during Dad's senior year of high school left my grandfather with two broken arms. That meant Dad had to start working to help his parents pay the bills. He spent some of that hard-earned money on toys too, buying a '69 Camaro convertible—white with red stripes—that was his pride and joy. He'd drive it around Senatobia and hang out at the Mug 'N Cone Drive-in with the other teenagers. That's where he met my mom, Elaine. She was a beauty, working on her cosmetology degree at Northwest Mississippi Community College, just across the street from the hangout.

Worried about being drafted into the Marines and sent to the front lines, Dad joined the Air Force with some buddies. He served a tour in Vietnam, came home to marry Mom, then went back for another. But when her health declined, the Air Force sent him home for good. An honorable discharge as his duty now was taking care of her. Then came my sister, Lori. Then me. And less than ten months later, my younger brother, Shannon.

When Lori was born, my parents lived in a single-wide trailer, moving it from place to place as Dad worked his way up the ladder at

Goodyear Tire. They lived in Booneville for a while, but that was too far away in my Nanny's opinion for her boy to live with his young family, so they moved to Amory, pulling that trailer behind them. That's where I was born. After Shannon came along, opportunity pulled them back to Strayhorn, Dad's hometown, where to Nanny's delight, they built a house just a few miles from her.

When my parents moved back, they bought one of those Jim Walters homes—the pre-manufactured "shell" houses people could finance with their land and finish out themselves. It was an affordable way to own a home, but it carried some of the same social stigma as a trailer. Still, my parents wanted a step up from that trailer they'd lived in as newlyweds, and this was it. To make it feel more like a "real" house, Dad had a friend help him put as much brick around the outside as they could afford. That was my childhood home, where I lived until high school.

I know Dad tried to do everything he could to make us feel comfortable, and for the most part, he did. Many of the decisions he made included that awareness. From the place we lived in to the town he moved us to. Growing up there gave me probably the best childhood a kid could have. The kind they used to have—ripping and running, riding dirt bikes, playing baseball with friends. No social media, no phones. Just fishing and hunting. True country-boy stuff. We never got into real trouble, but we did plenty of stupid stuff like BB gun fights—running through somebody's backyard taking potshots at each other. The only things that kept us from getting hurt were youth, bad aim, and dumb luck.

Our freedom didn't stop there. A group of five or six of us would ride our bikes down to the corner store, Mrs. Josephine's, to buy candy cigarettes and bubble gum that looked like chewing tobacco. We were trying to imitate the grown-ups, even if we'd never admit it. These were the people we loved and admired, like my Nanny, who always had a Virginia Slim between her fingers. But even though we had freedom, we knew we still had rules and knew to obey them. When the sun went down, playtime was over, and we had to get home for dinner. But that didn't mean the fun had to stop. At one point, that was one of my favorite parts of the day. It meant that I got to see my dad!

Us kids had to set the table every evening while Mom finished up in the kitchen. We all waited for him to get home and didn't eat until he'd walked through that door, cleaned up, and sat down. With five of us crowded around the table, it was always a toss-up who would get to sit next to him. I had my own way of making sure I won. As I set the table, I'd lick the back of the spoon at the place next to his. Lori and Shannon would gag and holler for Mom to make me stop, but they wouldn't touch it. That seat was mine.

Although we couldn't wait till Dad got home, he was strict. You'd better have cleaned your plate off, or else you would sit there until you did. Every last green pea or piece of broccoli down the hatch—no exceptions! That was just that generation's mentality. Many had grown up with parents who had lived through the Great Depression and had nothing. They learned to be grateful for every morsel their parents had given them. At the time we didn't know we were learning too; we were just obeying. Whether it was my favorite or a dish I dreaded, every bite was swallowed.

As is typical in the Bible Belt of the Southern U.S., we were raised in church. When I was a young boy, one Sunday my siblings and I were led out of the nursery into the sanctuary, where my parents were being baptized in the hand-painted baptismal of our little country church. We thought we were headed straight down to the Jordan River. We watched in awe as the pastor submerged each of them, then lifted them back up to clapping and *Amens* from the congregation. And then, just as matter-of-factly, the children's ministry volunteer led us right back to the nursery, as if we hadn't just witnessed something miraculous.

Some things changed dramatically after my parents' baptism. Dad became a music minister and even sang in a gospel quartet for a while. He also led Sunday school and the RAs—the missions training program for young boys in many Southern Baptist churches back then. We'd bow our heads to pray at dinner, but we never said what really needed saying. We would attend church on Sundays, but the sermons never seemed to affect our daily lives—at least not the way it did for Mom and Lori. For Dad and me, the same old demons kept torturing and tormenting under the surface, eager to lose the gag that had been placed on them.

DAD'S DRINKING began as nightly beers—his way of dealing with what Vietnam left behind. This infuriated the ladies at the church. Then, on top of that, their oldest boy got a girl pregnant before they were married. Let's just say that our family gave the church gossips something to talk about. But because of the stares and whispers, Mom couldn't take it anymore. She decided to move to a smaller congregation. Dad and I didn't follow. It gave us the excuse we needed to stop going altogether. Besides, after working six days a week, the last thing we wanted to do was spend half of our Sunday confined to a pew. Mom went to church, while he and I stayed home. Me with my friends, and him with his—the bottle.

"It helps me sleep boy," he would say. Dad had these terrible nightmares from Vietnam and would wake up back in the rice fields of the war. He would sleep with a knife in his hand to protect himself from imaginary foes. Mom would call either me or Shannon or both to come get him up, scared that he would wake up and attack her. He had made her promise that she would never try to wake him up, scared of the same thing she was—that he would view her as the enemy.

HE MOVED up the ranks at Goodyear Tire and everything seemed fine. He was doing good. Sharp dresser. Handshake firm as a vice. Customers liked him. He was the kind of man you'd want to buy something from. Back then, I was proud to say I was his son.

But the drinking wasn't just on the weekends. It was every day. And not just at night. It started showing up in his breath, in his temper, in the way his hands shook if he hadn't had any by lunch. One drink became six. Six became a bottle. Then it was a half-gallon every two or three days, sometimes faster.

He'd laugh too loud. Get real arrogant. Slur his words and talk over everybody like he was the smartest man in the room. But he wasn't. Not anymore.

You couldn't count on him. He'd say he'd pick you up or be somewhere—and then he just wouldn't show. Or he'd show up drunk. Too drunk to help. Too drunk to care. That was the part that stung the most. I got in a wreck on the way to school one day. Someone sideswiped me. I was seventeen and knew I couldn't call my dad or he would show up drunk and make matters worse. So I handled it alone.

As I got older, the drinking that was confined to a family problem began to affect others. He got DUIs. He would work at the shop all day, then drink all evening, and then drive home drunk. One night, he hit a lady. Got arrested. Hadn't been the first time I had to go bail him out of jail, and it wouldn't be the last. You start to wonder if the bottle meant more to him than you did.

IT DIDN'T HAPPEN ALL AT ONCE. That's the thing about it. It creeps up quiet. Like a thief. By the time I was a senior in high school, I wasn't just watching it—I was living with the wreckage.

Graduation came on a warm May night, the air thick with honeysuckle and sweat. My mom cried, of course. She'd gotten me through school, and now I was a high school graduate. Dad was proud too—said it more than once.

He asked what we had planned after the ceremony, and I told him straight: big field party out at a buddy's place. We would all climb in our trucks and cars with what booze we could get someone to buy and head to the country field with coolers full of cheap beer and build a bonfire. That's how we did it in Mississippi. No fancy dinners. Just friends, music, and the kind of drinking that made you feel grown.

Dad lit up when I told him. Said, "Wait right here." He came back with a trunk full of champagne and wine—top shelf stuff. "All for you and the boys. Don't leave the field, though," he said. "You stay put." And we did. To my friends, I was a legend. The guy whose dad brought the party. They all thought he was the coolest. Truth be told, I thought so too—for about five minutes.

But even then, something didn't sit right.

I kept one eye on his cooler and the other on him. He was already slurring before the sun went down. Didn't take much to guess he'd been drinking since lunch. When he pulled away from that field, his tires kicked up more dirt than a tractor, and his taillights swerved like they couldn't make up their mind.

Folks laughed. Said, "Man, your old man knows how to have a good time." But I didn't laugh. My stomach turned. I felt hot all over, like I'd swallowed the bonfire burning in the field. I didn't stop the party. I drank the champagne. I laughed too loud and acted like it didn't bother me. But somewhere in the back of my mind, I saw a future I didn't want. A man I didn't want to become.

I didn't know it yet, but that night marked a turning point. That was the start of me seeing things differently. What looked like fun from the outside started to feel more like something cracked open. Like something broke.

I TURNED my head ever so slightly in my hospital bed, trying to point my eyes in my parents' direction, trying to see through the bandages which of those demons was tormenting them now as they held vigil, praying their boy would live long enough to face his own.

## 6

# THE BUSINESSMAN

As days crawled by, I went from hearing people say, *"He might not make it through the night,"* to *"We don't know how he's still alive."* And in that strange limbo, I'd scribble on the pad, "Store?" asking Travis how things were going. Travis McDonald visited often. He also helped Dad and Bill keep the store running while I stayed stuck in that in-between place—burning but alive, with no one knowing for how long. I couldn't keep my thoughts from drifting to my store. I wasn't just the owner—I ran the place. Sales, management, all of it. It was what kept my family, and those that counted on me, fed and clothed, and well taken care of. Not being there felt almost as terrifying as the doctors not knowing if I'd live.

"Don't worry about it, man," Travis would say. "We've got this. You just focus on getting well enough to leave this place."

He meant it to be reassuring. But it didn't land that way.

Could I really trust Dad to run the store, the same store that was supposed to be his legacy, and mine? I thought of the trust I asked of those that I had rescued from fires, "Take my hand, I will get you out." Yet, I felt unable to trust my own father when it was my fate hanging in the balance. Maybe it would've been easier to trust a stranger. Maybe the problem was that I knew him all too well. The silence in the room allowed me to think. *How is it possible that somebody can be both a stranger and familiar at the same time?*

Maybe I was being too hard on him. After all, Dad had been a savvy businessman. He started with little but was determined to give us more. He'd do whatever he could to make sure we had everything we wanted—within reason, of course. When credit lines became a thing, letting people pay things out over twelve months, he bought my brother and me motorcycles. Little Honda 80s. We'd ride them for hours, no helmets, no cell phones—just gone. More freedom than we had any business having. Nothing like what we'd ever allow our own kids.

I had idolized my dad. He was a hard worker who had worked his way up from tire changer to district manager, a position that required driving up to twelve hours a day. Yet, despite all his traveling, I remember him being at my little league games, and walking into the house most nights late, but just in time to eat before shooing us kids to bed.

Then, when I was between ninth and tenth grade, my parents made a lot of big changes in a short amount of time. Dad decided he was done with all the travel. Said it wasn't what he needed to be doing anymore which was probably a blessing because when Dad started traveling for work, he started drinking. Socializing and meeting with clients went hand in hand with alcohol. They were almost inseparable—steak dinners, cocktails, wine with the meal, more drinks afterward—it was the perfect environment to feed those demons from Vietnam that came back to haunt him.

I'd always seen him as strong. Steady. But the drinking changed that. He stopped making it home for dinner. Didn't answer the phone when you needed a ride. Wobbled a little when he walked in at night. The bottle of liquor was his crutch, and he leaned on it hard.

Regardless of the reasons, or possibly marital threats, that brought it about, Dad cashed in on all he learned from climbing the ranks at Goodyear, and bought the tire store in Senatobia. For the family, owning the business meant moving into town. Bigger house, better schools. But being in Senatobia, we were still close enough to keep Nanny happy. Lori, my older sister, was about to start her senior year, but the move wasn't a big deal for her—her friends were in Senatobia, and her boyfriend went to school in town. Shannon was heading into ninth grade, so he had to switch schools anyway. I was the one who felt the move the most.

Dad saw Senatobia Tire as a legacy, something to pass down to me and Shannon. I don't know if either of us thought about it much, but to him, it was everything. For a country boy with nothing more than a high school diploma, being a business owner was a big deal. My Nanny was proud as could be. Owning a business meant something. It wasn't just a paycheck; it was proof. Proof that hard work could take you places. Proof that her son had built something from the ground up. That the American Dream was alive and well, and that Nanny's son was living it.

WHEN WE MOVED TO TOWN, I sat beside Dad in the front office of the new school, slouched in the hard plastic chair, staring at a crack in the tile. I already knew this wasn't gonna be a pep talk. I was staring at the very real possibility of having to repeat ninth grade and being in class with my younger brother. I hated school. The factory model of the late '80s—where kids sat in quiet rows, filling out endless worksheets—drove my hyperactive attention crazy. I wasn't a troublemaker, but sitting still at a desk for eight hours a day? Impossible. I wanted to be up and active, hands-on. Show me, let me do it, and I'd pick it up no problem. Make me sit still and listen to a teacher drone on? No way. Thus, the vo-tech classes that I had taken were okay. Algebra? I still don't see the point. Thus, it hadn't been long before my inability to fit inside the classroom mold started catching up with me.

Across from us, the school administrator flipped through my file, lips pursed like he was chewing on a decision.

Dad didn't wait for him to say much. "Look," he said, leaning forward with his arms on his knees. "He ain't gonna be a doctor. He's gonna come work for me at the Tire Store. So let's not act like he's headed to college on a scholarship."

The administrator blinked. I did too.

Not that I had ever shied away from hard work. At twelve years old, I'd drive myself around the neighborhood in Dad's truck with a little push mower. Nobody questioned it, not even the local cops, who were also my customers. One old man had grinned while handing me twenty dollars in cash for the lawn I had just finished mowing.

"That's some work ethic you got there boy. What do you plan to do when you grow up?"

I had dusted my hands on my jeans. "Get my own truck. I would love a fishing boat, too."

The old man laughed, "No, son. I mean a career. What do you plan on doing with yourself?"

"Working, sir, and making money." He just shook his head.

"Ok, boy, well you do that."

I wasn't chasing some big dream or flashy career. I didn't care what the job was, as long as it paid well and left time for me to enjoy myself.

Dad went on. "I'm not askin' you to give him a pass. Just get him through this. Give him what he needs to graduate and get to work."

The man nodded slowly, then looked at me. "That what you want?"

I shrugged. "Yeah. I just don't wanna get held back. I can't be in class with Shannon as his older brother. That would be humiliating." That seemed to amuse Dad more than anything I'd said all year.

They laid out a plan right there of what I had to do to graduate. I'd have to double up and finish both ninth and tenth grade in one shot. It was gonna be tough, but I would force myself to do it. It was better than the alternative. I could do anything I set my mind to; I just needed a good motivator, and staying a grade ahead of my younger brother was a big one.

. . .

Working for Dad at the Tire Store is exactly what I did. I always had a nice truck, hunting gear, a boat, and long Sundays to enjoy the toys I had worked so hard for. It also allowed me to pick up the slack and prevent business from suffering when Dad took his long lunches and had nobody to run the floor.

By the time I was 24, Dad was ready to retire. Bill Weeks and I bought the Goodyear store from him, which meant I never really worked for anybody but myself. We also started a dirt work company —land clearing, excavation, laying foundations, building houses. Everything we touched made money, but we earned it. Worked six, sometimes seven days a week.

I didn't believe in hoarding money away for some possible future. I believed in using it now to improve life today. If a car didn't suit me, or I found one I liked better, I would sell the old one and get a new one. We sold our first house and bought a second, not far from the first. I wasn't just providing. I wanted to prove something. Prove that I could give my family the best. I wasn't just getting by; I was thriving, and it felt good.

It felt good to take care of the people I loved. I'd take my buddies to the steakhouse and cover the tab for ten ribeyes without even blinking. When my brother-in-law, Clark, couldn't leave base to drive Lori and their girls home for Christmas, I bought her plane tickets so they could fly in and spend time with Mom and Dad—and her in-laws, too. That's what money is for—helping others. It's for spoiling your loved ones, and maybe yourself, too, when you can.

But being the store owner didn't mean I just made the big bucks; it meant I had flexibility. I could take fire calls whenever I wanted to, and I wanted to every time that pager went off. But now, lying here in this hospital bed, wired up and broken, all I could think about was the store, the fires, and *Please, Dad, don't destroy what you and I built.*

# 7

## THE BROTHER

Days stretched to weeks, and I was still in the hospital. There were friends who sent their love and support, and then there were brothers. A brother by blood who paced up and down the hospital corridors and drove Mom, Dad, and Chrissi wherever they needed to go. Brother by marriage, off fighting a war on terror while I fought the terror inside me. Brothers on the force, who showed up to the hospital in such numbers that makeshift waiting rooms had to be opened to hold them all. And friends who had become brothers who were the heartbeat that kept all of us going, fighting to make it through one more day.

When the pain got bad and the hours felt like days, I'd drift. Not asleep. Not really awake. Just somewhere else. They say your mind does that when the body's had enough. Finds a place it remembers feeling whole. For me, that place was with my brothers.

I HAD BEEN at Senatobia High School when I met Jimmie Neal and Zander Billingsley. For over a decade, we had been thick as thieves. We stood in each other's weddings, became firefighters together, raised our kids side by side, and walked through all the highs and lows of growing up.

We bonded over our shared love of the outdoors, with pickup trucks replacing the dirt bikes of our youth. Shannon and I used to ride together to school in the mornings. It became routine—he would slide into the passenger seat, and I would slide my shotgun on the rack in the back window of my truck. Nobody thought twice about those guns in our trucks. Back then, a shotgun in a country boy's truck at school was normal.

"Hey, man, you ready to get that buck we saw yesterday?" I called to Jimmie as we pulled up next to him in the parking lot.

"Not if you scare it off again," he shot back over the hood.

We slung our backpacks on and walked towards the long cement building.

"You boys have any luck this weekend," the principal called to us, nodding towards our trucks.

"Yes, sir," I said. "Got a nice doe. She's gonna make some good chili. You?"

He grinned. "Not yet, heading back out Saturday" he said, already turning to the next wave of kids filing in.

As I moved into adulthood, the group just kept growing. I added more friends, like Travis McDonald and Bill Weeks. Travis was a big guy with an even bigger heart—everybody called him "Big Trav." Bill was the life of the party, always talkative and ready to turn anybody into his next best friend.

Before long, we had a whole crew that stuck together most weekends, especially in the summer. Bill had a ski boat, I had a pontoon, and my brother had the jet skis. We'd load up the wives and kids, coolers full of burgers, steaks, hot dogs, and plenty to drink, and head out to Sardis Lake. There was this little cove we claimed as our spot—made it our home base on the water. I had a small grill on my boat, and we'd fire it up while Bill pulled the kids behind his boat on inner tubes and kneeboards. The jet skis would zoom by, throwing up wakes that launched the kids into the air, which they thought was the greatest thing ever—even if it about gave their mamas a heart attack.

We'd stay out there all day, coming home sunburned, worn out, and happy. Some weekends, we'd throw tents or campers into the mix and not come home until late Sunday night—just in time to get the kids to bed and drag ourselves to work the next morning.

We didn't go to church much; we spent Sundays with friends. Church was more of a social ritual I had little use for than a means of my faith. Not that we didn't believe in God, but my dad's baptism had not really changed him. It changed some of his outward behavior for a time, sure, but his inner demons were still ever-present. The drinking stole away any trust I had in him to be sober when it counted. This circle of friends that I surrounded myself with—those that showed up every weekend and answered my calls in the middle of the night when I needed them most—that was the social circle I wanted to be with on Sundays.

WE HAD a pool put in at the house on Yellow Dog Road, turning Sundays spent on the lake to all-day get-togethers at our place. Everybody would show up, and I'd fire up the grill. The kids splashed in the bright blue water while the wives kicked back in chairs lined with beach towels, laughing and catching up.

We had a sunroom that looked out over the pool with windows all along the back wall. I'd put in Mexican tile floors so we didn't have to worry about wet feet messing up wood or carpet. We added a pool table too, and that's where the guys usually hung out, cue sticks in hand, taking turns beating each other while we waited on the burgers to be done.

When our days at the lake became days around the pool, I looked at Chrissi one hot afternoon and said, "Well, I guess we can sell the boat now. No need to haul off to the lake when we've got this in the backyard." But the kids overheard me and weren't having it.

"You can't sell the boat!" they said. "The lake and the pool aren't the same thing, Dad!"

They were right. So we kept the boat. And the camper. And all the toys that made busting it all week worth it when Friday rolled around.

OUR GROUP of friends loved hanging out together so much, we would take a weeklong trip together, just the adults, to Arkansas every summer where we would float down the river and eat too much, laugh too loud, and for those that wanted, drink too much. We were a pack, and we traveled like it.

We also knew how to talk to each other, tell each other the truth even when we didn't want to hear it. And there were times I definitely didn't want to hear it. We would get mad at each other, not talk for a while, then finally one of us would break and call, and we would be back as if nothing ever happened.

BUT I DIDN'T ALLOW myself to think about the hard times, not in the hospital. There, I had to focus on what the doctors said would get me out of here. Like the doctor that came in one morning.

"Pat," he said, his chair scraped across the floor to the edge of my bed, "we need to go ahead with a tracheotomy."

I scribbled on my small dry-erase board, "Why?"

"The skin around your mouth is closing in," he said. "That small opening you've got now? It's disappearing. Right now, we can still get a straw in. But at this rate, eventually it would get too small to intubate for surgeries.

I let that sink in. I already hated the tubes. Every time they shoved one in, they had to rip my mouth open all over again. It felt like knives.

"It's just too risky to keep damaging the skin around your mouth," he added. "Too traumatic. This will make it safer. And it'll make the next steps easier."

Didn't like it. Didn't want it. But I understood.

Later, after the procedure, they capped it—said I'd be able to talk some. Not a lot, but enough.

It wasn't much. But in that moment, it felt like something was being handed back to me instead of being taken away from me. I needed that.

But there always seemed to be a price to pay for every step forward. In this case, it was the thick, nasty mess they made me swallow to help coat my throat. Make it easier to swallow, get the muscles working again after the trach. I tried to drink it and gagged. It was awful, like a mixture of glue and snot.

The little PT kid kept pushing.

"You have to try," he said. His voice all polite and peppy, like I was a toddler refusing broccoli.

He didn't know who he was dealin' with.

"Nope," I told him, my voice a raspy whisper that was the opposite of the loud determination I felt.

"It's important." He said, as if that solved all my objections.

"I don't care."

He put the straw up to my lips again. I pulled it away.

Then I slung it across the room. Hard. My throwing arm from baseball still worked just fine.

It hit with a loud *thunk*.

"Everything okay in here?" A female voice called from across the room—a nurse checking to see what had happened.

"Yea, yeah. It's fine." The kid stammered.

Bill was in the corner, flipping through a magazine. "Alright," he said. "Give us a minute."

"Uh..."

"Just five minutes," Bill said. "Go."

I heard the door shut.

"You listenin'?" he said. "Cause I'm only gonna say this once."

I didn't move.

I heard his footsteps as he walked over and sat in the chair beside the bed.

"These people? They don't have to care. But they do. They're here 24/7, wipin' you, cleanin' you, tryin' to get you back on your feet."

He wasn't raising his voice. That's how I knew he was serious.

"You don't want 'em here? Guess what? They don't wanna be here either. But they *are*. Because they believe you're worth it."

I didn't respond.

"You've been in and out for a month, Pat. A whole stretch of your life. And while you were gone, these folks learned how to keep you alive. Now it's your turn. You gotta learn how to *live* again."

His voice was closer to me now.

"I know it hurts. I know it all sucks. But you've come too far to start actin' like a child over a cup of thick goop."

I didn't say anything.

But when the kid came back in, fresh cup in hand, I drank it.

Still tasted repulsive.

But I got it down.

Without throwing anything.

Like I said, we were brothers. We didn't sugarcoat things. We told each other the truth, even when it stung. Because that is when it is most important. And usually, we didn't want to listen. But we heard.

That day, I heard him.

## 8

## THE HUSBAND

I felt a familiar hand slide across the rough hospital blanket and close around mine. I turned toward her instinctively. My partner. My wife. The mother of my children. Chrissi. A month in and she was still here, holding my hand.

Many times in those early days, she was my comfort, and the only thing that would calm me when the nightmares wouldn't quit. The nurses would go find her and ask her to come to the room, even though it was between visiting hours.

"Pat woke up and is really agitated. Looks like he had a nightmare again. Can you come see if you can calm him down?" And she would. Something about her calm and confident voice telling me we were going to make it through did the trick. She would assure me I wasn't in the fire anymore.

WE SAY THOSE VOWS—*IN sickness and in health*—and we mean them. Or we think we do. But when you're young and in love, those words sound more like poetry than a promise. You equate that to maybe a flu or possibly a surgery one day when you're old and gray. You don't picture *this*.

You don't picture feeding your husband through a straw. Sleeping in a stiff hospital chair night after night. Changing bandages—or worse, diapers—on the man you once made love to.

WE'D ONLY BEEN MARRIED three years. Just long enough to start settling into the reality of it all. Long enough to roll over one morning and realize, *Oh, you're actually going to be here every day for the rest of my life.*

Just long enough for the cute little things—like the way she tapped her fork on her plate—to start getting on my nerves. Those things were almost expected—the common growing pains of marriage. But this?

We hadn't signed up for this. Not this level of sickness. Not this level of sacrifice. Our vows were being tested far beyond what most people ever face.

Or I should say—*her* vows were.

Being the one who is in the hospital is hard, no doubt. But it's not the same as being the one who stays. The one who keeps it all running. The bills. The kids. The house. Then add nurse, maid, scheduler, chauffeur, and caretaker to the list.

It's not sexy. It's not romantic. This is where the rubber meets the road, and you find out if you're going to hold to those vows.

When you're the patient, no one expects you to hold it together. But the caregiver? They don't get the same grace.

Her load tripled overnight—and she was expected to carry it without question, without complaint, and without ever putting it down.

THIS WASN'T the first time the vows I had made in a marriage were tested. My oldest daughter, Alison, wasn't even two when my first wife, Rebecca, and I divorced. We admitted to ourselves that it wasn't working between us and went our separate ways.

I prayed a lot then, asking God what we were doing this for. Truth was, I never really wanted a divorce, but our hearts weren't in the marriage. What else could we do? Lying to ourselves that things were going to get better was only making it worse. We both knew we'd be happier apart. Only thing I never regretted was our daughter.

Divorce didn't feel like freedom at first; it felt like failure. Not just in a marriage sense, but like I'd let everybody down—my family, her family, Alison, society, the church. I wasn't the kind of man who quit. But sometimes persistence is more punishment than it is perseverance. We had to finally accept that the pieces just didn't fit.

IRONICALLY, it was Rebecca's cousin who had called me one night, with a plan to get me back on my dating feet. "Hey, Pat," she said, "got somebody you need to meet. I thought maybe you could drop by my house tomorrow night for supper and I would introduce y'all."

I raised an eyebrow. "Oh yeah?"

"Yeah. Her name is Chrissi and she is a good friend of mine. She just got out of a relationship, and I think y'all would really hit it off. Got a little baby boy. Sweet as they come."

"Yeah, OK, why not." I told her. I figured I didn't have anything to lose, and who knows, maybe we would hit it off. And she was right. We did.

At first, it was simple—low-key hangouts at my house or down at the deer camp. I'd cook dinner, or we'd swing through the Sonic and get a couple of burgers. She had her son with her, and I had Alison with me, so there was always a kid around. We'd let down the back of the truck, watch the kids play on the swings at the park, and just talk. There was no performance with her. No pressure to be anything fancy.

She laughed easily. That stood out. Chrissi didn't need big dates or perfect plans. She just wanted to be together. She loved Dalton the way I loved Alison, and I saw the way she looked at both kids like they were gifts, not burdens. That stuck with me. She treated my daughter like her own before she had any reason to.

Before long, we were inseparable. The kind of togetherness where her toothbrush lived at my place and mine ended up at hers. The kind where it just made sense. We got married, and I adopted Dalton. I am not sure who I fell in love with first, her or him. Then, we had Averi, the first of our children together. I always said I wanted a big family—ten kids if I could. That was before I realized how expensive they were. Kids don't just eat food—they eat time, money, patience, gas, and the last cookie in the house. But man, I loved being a dad.

IN 1999, Chrissi and I bought twenty acres and a house out on Yellow Dog Road, not far from my parents. It was our dream place. Truth was, we didn't love the house—but we loved the land. Loved the spot. It felt like ours. Like something we could build on. You can always fix up a house, but you can't move a perfect piece of land.

I wanted Chrissi to make it exactly what she wanted. Something just right for her and the kids. I'd watched my dad take a plain old house and turn it into a home for us growing up, and I wanted to do that for her. Give her something she could be proud of. A place where we could grow old together. A home that would hold our family's story.

Some nights, after the kids were in bed, we'd sit out on the porch —just the two of us and the crickets. I'd watch the sun drop behind the pines and feel that deep-down peace you can't buy. *I built this*, I thought. Not just the house, but the life inside it. And it felt good.

Most people saw the house with the pool, the nice cars, the boat, the toys—and thought we had it easy. What they didn't see was me up before daylight, not coming in till dark. Chrissi holding down the house and raising our babies while I worked.

But together? We had been building something that mattered. Something we had hoped to pass down—just like my dad had done with the store.

BUT IN THAT HOSPITAL ROOM, as we sat there in silence holding hands, it felt like the life we'd spent the last three years building was coming apart around us.

Mom stuck her head in the room. "You ready?" she asked Chrissi.

Our eyes met briefly before she looked over at Mom and nodded. "I told my sister I would be there in time to have dinner with the kids. I have to get a few bills paid and pack a fresh bag before I head back this way. She told me she did the laundry, so I don't have to worry about that. Shannon said he would mow the yard tomorrow after he got home from work."

"Honey don't rush back," Mom said, "That's a 45-minute drive. It will be after 11 tonight before you get back up here. I can get Ed to come up and stay with me tonight. You sleep in your own bed for a change."

"No, I need to get back here," Chrissi insisted. "They are doing another procedure in the morning. I took a nap earlier." Mom huffed at the notion that a nap in a chair at my bedside had given her any sort of rest.

Stuck in this hospital, the yard didn't get mowed by me. The housework didn't get done by her. Meals were usually grabbed from the hospital cafeteria—whatever was quick. The rhythm of our lives was just... gone.

No Saturdays by the pool. No weekends at the lake. No dinners with friends or messy Tuesday nights with toddlers in highchairs and toys underfoot.

Instead, there were phone calls to say goodnight from another state. Short visits that always ended too soon. Days filled with doctors, nurses, diagnoses, prognoses and one question after another about what came next.

Would I ever be well enough to come home?

Would I ever work again?

And maybe hardest of all—

Would Chrissi ever get to be anything more than my caretaker?

WHAT MOST PEOPLE don't understand—unless they've lived through it—is just how much *work* comes with a long hospital stay. It's not just sitting by a bed, holding someone's hand, praying they'll get better. It's a full-time job.

There's the paperwork. Mountains of it. Insurance claims. Worker's comp. Social workers with clipboards and questions. Rehab facilities calling to "coordinate care." Nurses that change every twelve hours. Dozens of doctors rotating through—each with their own opinion, each speaking a language you've got to learn fast. Medications. Schedules. Risks. Side effects.

And just when you've memorized one set of meds, they change it again.

That's inside the hospital. Outside? Life keeps coming. The mortgage still needs to be paid. So do the lights, the water, the car insurance. If the paychecks stop, that means more paperwork—more hold music, more explaining why you're late, why you need more time.

And then, in our case, there was the media. Reporters calling for comment. News vans outside. Lawyers wanting to sue the city, the fire department, the homeowners, the hospital—anyone they think might write a check.

But none of them could talk to me. I was barely conscious.

So, it all landed on Chrissi dealing with all of this while barely being able to get a comfortable rest.


AND HERE'S what they *really* don't tell you: Where was she expected to *relax and catch up on rest* when her husband is in a tightly controlled environment with no extra bed, no recliner in the corner? In the middle of a busy urban trauma center waiting room where rival gang members sat across from each other. Next to families just waiting for word about their loved ones who had been in a car crash. No one from our family was willing to let her sit alone in that waiting room, much less leave her bags for a few minutes to come visit me.

It only took a day or two for the staff to notice. After seeing how rough it was on her and my mom, they finally stepped in. Maintenance cleared out an old closet, and someone dragged in a bed and a chair.

A CLOSET.

THAT'S where Chrissi lived for weeks. Sharing a single bed with my mom, taking turns sleeping and rotating to see me during visiting hours. Hiding from the reporters. From the chaos. From the danger. She walked in one time after sleeping in the closet, and I heard her voice, tired and hoarse. That feeling of being a failure from my first divorce crept back in. *I failed her. What did it matter that I bought us a house for her to be comfortable and sleep in a big bed? It was because of me now that she was sleeping in a closet.* I had to get out of this hospital bed and provide for her again. Show her I was still the man she once married.

# 9

## THE DAD

One month turned into two. And I still hadn't seen my kids. Who wants their children to see that? The tubes. The burns. The smell of infection and chemicals. Machines that beeped and hissed like something out of a horror movie.

Chrissi and Rebecca had agreed: the kids wouldn't come until I was almost ready to go home. They'd been told I was hurt in a fire. Told I'd come home—but it would take a while. Then told I wouldn't look like the dad they remembered. We tried to prepare them. But how do you prepare a child for their dad leaving one morning looking just like he always had…and coming home months later with a face burned beyond recognition?

Being a dad was one of the greatest joys of my life. And I hadn't seen my babies for two months.

I missed their voices. Their hugs. The sound of three pairs of little bare feet running through the house. I missed hollering at them to come to dinner, helping cut up meat and veggies into toddler-sized portions, helping them down from their highchairs so they could go tearing off, back into their make-believe world.

The doctors were finally saying I was strong enough to go home. I couldn't wait. Yet, I had one more hurdle to overcome before I left—

seeing the kids, or should I say, allowing the kids to see me. As Chrissi sat next to my bed, laying out the plans for how I would finally get to hold my babies, my mind wondered back, to learning my oldest was on the way, and telling my parents I was going to be a dad.

I DON'T REMEMBER WALKING into the kitchen that evening, but I remember standing there in front of my parents—heart pounding, hands clenching and unclenching.

"I gotta tell you something," I said.

Mom's eyes locked on mine. "What is it?"

I didn't try to ease into it. No small talk. No buildup.

"Rebecca's pregnant."

Silence.

Mom didn't yell. She didn't cry. She just sat there a second, then placed her hands in her lap real slow. Her voice was calm. Flat. The kind of calm that meant there would be no changing her mind. "You're not gonna embarrass this family like that," she said. Then, without missing a beat, "You and Rebecca are getting married. Now." There wasn't a question mark at the end of that sentence.

I didn't argue. Not because I was ready—but because I already knew. That's just how things worked in a town like ours. You didn't get a girl pregnant and then see what happened next.

Mom stood up, already shifting into planning mode. "You two were talking about getting married in the fall—we'll just move it up a few months." She headed out of the kitchen, to get paper and pen and get started.

I walked out on shaky legs, grateful that there had not been a confrontation, just a simple statement of fact. I had gone in as somebody's teenage son. I walked out as a soon-to-be husband and father.

NOW I WOULD HAVE three people all depending on me. I had the job at the tire store, so I didn't figure providing for a family would be that much of a stretch. I had found one thing that I was really good at—sales. Some guy would come in needing to get a plug put in a tire and leave with a new set of rims. Life was good, and there was lots of money to be made for someone good at selling, and apparently, I was. Turns out, I could talk just about anybody into buying just about anything.

Before the wedding, Rebecca and I started looking for houses, found one we liked, but learned that it wasn't as easy as just putting up the down payment and signing the papers.

"What do you mean I can't buy it?" I said into the phone, fighting to keep my voice even and controlled.

"Well, you aren't twenty-one yet, Pat. I assumed your Dad would be signing for the house for you. You can't buy a house as a minor." The banker explained.

"What do you mean, "a minor"? I have a full-time job, am about to be married, and a kid on the way. In what world am I a minor that needs his daddy to sign for him to buy a house?"

"Mississippi," he said.

I couldn't buy it. But that wasn't gonna work for me. Don't tell me I can't do something. "You can't complete two years of high school in one year, Pat. You already about failed your first year." But I completed them. "You can't drive around here mowing yards, you are only twelve years old." But I drove. And I would figure out a way to do this, too.

The next Sunday at church, I cornered a local realtor. "Hey, Ann, apparently I am too young to buy house."

"What?" She asked, glancing back at the ladies she had been visiting with as if to say this wouldn't take but a second.

"Yep. Bank says I can't buy that house I want to get for me and Rebecca until I am twenty-one. Surely there has to be a way around this."

She pursed her lips for a second. "You know, there just might be. You could go to the judge and ask him to remove your minority, you know, given your special circumstances. He issues you an order making you an adult in the eyes of the law. Then, you can do anything a twenty-one-year-old can—well, except drink. You still have to be old enough for that, Pat."

"I ain't worried about drinking, I'm worried I won't have a house to bring my baby home. Can you help me do this?"

"Why, sure, I can do that. Come by tomorrow and we will call the judge and see what all you need to bring him."

And just like that, I went to the local judge, explained the situation, and with a signature on a few pieces of paper, I was no longer a minor in the eyes of the law. Mississippi was now willing to let me take out a loan on a house, with the only difference being a judge agreed I was old enough. I wasn't a kid figuring things out. I was a dad with mouths to feed. I told myself I was ready. Maybe I even believed it. But a part of me still felt like that kid on his dirt bike, wearing grown-up shoes and playing house with the girl down the street.

AFTER REBECCA AND I DIVORCED, and I married Chrissi, I wanted to provide for her son as much as I could. So, I adopted Dalton. Now, I had one of each. But God wasn't done with giving me kids. The year after Chrissi and I married, we had a child of our own, Averi—a beautiful little bundle of blonde hair and blue eyes. I was a dad of three under the age of five before I was half-way to thirty. I'd wake up before the kids, brush my teeth while the coffee brewed in the kitchen. Chrissi would get the kids up one by one, hair sticking up, pajamas twisted from sleep. I'd ruffle heads, pour cereal, sip my coffee while trying not to step on stray toys.

We had birthday parties in the backyard—bounce houses, balloons, cake smudged on cheeks. Halloween meant plastic pumpkins and costumes picked out weeks in advance. I was the dad pulling a wagon down the sidewalk while Chrissi walked beside the kids, reminding them to say thank you at every door.

Christmas Eve? That was my shift. Once the kids were asleep, I'd be out in the shop with a screwdriver and a cold Coke, piecing together dollhouses and racetracks under the hum of a work light. One year, I thought I would get a head start and do it at the tire store between customers. Christmas was slow, with everyone spending money on presents instead of tires. So I got to the shop and started the coffee and began laying out all the toys that needed to be put together. That's when Travis called.

"Hey, man, I won't be in today, I'm real sick."

"What do you mean you're sick? Look, I'm swamped up here today, I really need your help. If you can make it at all, I would really appreciate it." It had been partially true, at least.

"OK, I'll be there as soon as I can."

But when he walked in and saw that the store was dead and the help I wanted was for him to play Elf to my Santa, not sell tires, he just chuckled. "You have got to be kidding me!" But he wasn't mad, just grabbed a hot cup of coffee and a screwdriver and got to work. Became a tradition. He would come and help put the toys together every year, sometimes even bringing extra recruits. We would be up until three or four in the morning, every toy I purchased seemingly coming with a million parts that needed to be put together.

WE TAUGHT them how to swim in the backyard pool—me in the water, arms outstretched, calling for them to let go of the edge and jump to me. I ran behind their bikes on the driveway, hand steady on the seat until they found their balance and took off on their own.

And when I needed to breathe, we'd jump on the four-wheeler. Just me and one of the kids on my lap, fingers wrapped around the handlebars. We'd ride slow through the woods behind the house, and I'd point things out as we went—deer tracks in the mud, the bend in the creek, a tree that looked like it had a face if you tilted your head just right.

AND THEN, for sixty-three days in 2001, I didn't see them. Not once. No messy hair in the mornings. No little voices calling out for Daddy. No Halloween costumes or bike rides or tiny hands reaching for mine.

Just a hospital bed. Machines. Pain.

And the silence where their laughter used to be.

THE FIRST TIME the doctors mentioned sending me home, I was ecstatic! Chrissi started crying. I thought at first it was because she was as happy as I was to be going home to our kids.

"No, Pat. I'm scared. What am I going to do? I don't know how to give you your medicine or change these bandages. You have skin grafts over your eyes and can't even see! You have had nurses around the clock for months, and the idea of it just being me scares me more than when I brought Dalton home for the first time. At least then, I had taken care of a baby before. I've never done any of this. And we have to bring the kids up and let them see you. We don't know how they are going to respond to seeing you. I don't want them freaking out when you get home."

Her words brought me back down quick. This wasn't going to be an easy transition back to the life I had.

And so for the next few days, Chrissi got a crash course on nursing care. I had a feeding tube and a port-a-cath in my chest that they taught her how to care for. Sent her home with boxes of glass bottles full of antibiotics. They showed her how to hook up the bottles to my port, how to let the suction draw the meds in slow and steady. She'd sit with me while it ran, watching every drip. Didn't matter that she wasn't a nurse—she became one real quick.

THEN, a few days before I was released from the hospital, Chrissi led our two younger kids through the hospital corridors to see their bandage covered dad. The nurse had put me in a waiting room type area with a chair, where I could visit with them and not be in a hospital room. Dalton was hesitant for only a moment before jumping onto my lap. Chrissi cautioned him to be careful with the lines and tubes. Averi was a different story, however. She screamed a soul-piercing screech. The monster that was sitting in front of her with arms outstretched was trying to get her. Dalton scoffed, "It's just

Dad! What's wrong with you?" But she refused to come near the monster that she saw before her. It broke my heart that my precious little girl, one that just two months before would have run out of her room and into my arms as I came home for dinner, was refusing to come near me. Chrissi had to lead her out of the room while I visited with Dalton for the few minutes that I had. I tried to act brave while I died a little inside.

I DON'T REMEMBER MUCH about the ride home from the hospital. Bill and Chrissi loaded me up in the front passenger seat of the van and Bill drove while Chrissi sat in the back, boxes full of supplies on the seat next to her.

We got to Senatobia and Bill pulled into the gas station to get gas before the last little bit home. But when we pulled in, everybody just stopped—and stared. I should have realized then that this was how it was going to be for the rest of my life. But I didn't. Didn't see the stares, the skin grafts and bandages over my eyes hiding the awful truth from me. My life had completely changed—and everyone knew it but me.

# PART III
# THE MIRROR

## 10

## WHAT I SAW

People ask me all the time, "How did you survive that?"

And I tell them truthfully, "I don't know, God just pulled me through it. I never let myself think there was any other alternative."

Recovery isn't just physical. It's mental. Your body knows how to heal—it's built that way. With the right surgeries, meds, or just time, things mend if they can. But your mind? That's where the real fight happens.

The brain can do wild things. It can create pain that ain't there—or shut it off when it should be unbearable. It can convince you you're dying from a cold or keep you breathing when doctors are shaking their heads, wondering how you're still alive.

If you want to survive something like this, your mind has to decide first.

The Bible says He'll keep in perfect peace the one whose mind is stayed on Him. Mine was set—like concrete. Fireproof. I believed with everything in me that God was going to pull me through. Return me to the man I was before. That I wasn't going to die. That Chrissi wouldn't be left alone to raise our kids.

I didn't allow myself to think any differently.

. . .

AND I THINK about all the ways that God showed up, quietly in the background. Showed up before a single prayer had ever been uttered to save me, or heal me, or provide for us in the hour of our greatest need.

Like when this polished insurance saleslady sashayed into my office at the tire store late one afternoon, months before the accident.

"I'm here to see Pat Hardison," she said, sliding her business card across the counter.

I gave it a glance. "That's me. What's this about?"

"Do you mind if we go in your office and talk for a second?" She smiled and nodded towards the open office door behind me.

I almost said no. I had a lot to do. But something in her tone—or maybe just the way she was already walking around the counter—made me nod.

"Sure," I said against my better judgment, and motioned her into the office. "But I don't need insurance." I slid into my chair behind the desk.

"You have small children, don't you?" She pointed to the picture next to the computer monitor. "And you're a firefighter!" She pointed to a picture on the wall of me in my dress whites when I first joined the force. "You run into fires instead of away from them. Aren't you concerned about how your wife will care for those babies if the unthinkable happens? Our policies will cover you for various forms of catastrophic injuries, such as..." I stopped listening as she kept listing off every horrific injury you could imagine while sliding some brochures across the desk.

I cut her off without picking them up. "Look lady, I'm young and we are well trained. Been on the force six years. The store makes plenty of money, we'll be just fine with the insurance I already have."

"That's what everyone says until they are laying in ICU and their bills are going unpaid." She tilted her head and stared me down, as if daring me to argue.

I pulled off my ball cap, scratched my head as if searching for inspiration to get her out of my office and then put my hat back on. "OK, fine, what is your cheapest policy?"

"This one right here is what you need, only $12 per month and you can be covered today."

"Great. Here is a voided check." I tore one out of my checkbook in the top drawer and passed it across the desk to her. "Can we be done?"

She smiled and slid the check into her briefcase. "You won't regret this, Mr. Hardison." And she turned and sashayed right back out the front door. I felt like that was money well spent to get her to leave my office.

I wasn't worried about any injury, catastrophic or otherwise. Not that day. Not ever. I thought I was invincible.

Seven months later, what amounted to payments of $84 turned into a $300,000 insurance payout. It saved my family when neither Chrissi nor I could leave the hospital, much less work. Maybe she was an angel in disguise, maybe she was just good at sales, but either way, God sent her that day.

BUT WHEN I was in the hospital, awake enough to know I had indeed survived to face another day, I thought I'd be home in a couple of weeks. That's what I told myself. I didn't understand the damage, not really. I hadn't seen what the fire had done. No one had been able to show me a mirror and make me face the reality of what was going on. The grafts over my eyes prevented that. I had ignored the doctors when they discussed my recovery using words like "months" and "years." Didn't truly see the toll it was taking on everyone around me. I was 27 years old. A firefighter, a businessman, a son, a brother, a husband, and a dad. Our youngest was barely two. We owned our dream home. Life was great. How could one injury take any of that away from me? From us? We would make it. Chrissi, with the help of our friends and family, had been making sure everything stayed running. God had provided in the form of that miraculous insurance policy. I believed I was young and strong—uninjured from the shoulders down. As soon as we could get me home, I would go back to work and get us back on our feet. *Everything would be fine. These injuries were just superficial*, I thought.

Then I saw what had become of my head and face in that mirror that day as I passed by it on my way down the hall.

It wasn't the fire that broke me. It wasn't the surgeries. Wasn't the months of blindness or pain.

It was that mirror.

It should've shattered. Like in the fairy tales, where the monster looks in and the glass can't take it. But it didn't shatter. It stayed whole. I'm the one who broke. All of my dreams and plans for the future, all of my hope, shattered as surely as if I had punched that lying piece of glass.

I stared at the reflection. At the swollen skin, the patches of raw redness, the formless features that didn't belong to a human. My mind didn't try to soften the blow. It just screamed.

I looked at my dad standing behind me.

"If you love me, you'll go get my gun from the safe. Get Chrissi and the kids outta the house first. Then bring it to me."

That was when the dark began to close in.

# PART IV
# MY UNDOING

## 11

# HOME

The front door clicked shut behind us as Chrissi helped guide me inside, one arm under mine, the other grabbing the bag of gauze and bandages from the passenger seat.

"Watch the rug," she said softly, steering me around the edge of it so I wouldn't trip. My legs felt like wet noodles. My shoulders ached from the car ride. Memphis and back again—just like yesterday. Just like tomorrow.

The kids came running. "Mama! Mama! Look what I made!" Averi yelled, waving a construction paper mess in the air. Crayons everywhere. Glue still wet.

Chrissi gave her a tired smile. "That's beautiful, baby. Let me get Daddy settled and I will take a look."

She helped lower me into the recliner. I groaned as I sank back, every joint stiff, skin tugging under bandages that were already overdue for changing.

She was already in the kitchen before I could thank her. Cabinet doors opened. Oven creaked. The sound of a pot hitting the stovetop. The smell hit me quick—fried pork chops. The real kind, dredged in flour and pan-fried in Crisco. Potatoes bubbling in a pot. Biscuits going in the oven. I closed my eyes and breathed it in, slow and careful.

"Y'all wash up!" she hollered to the kids. Their feet pounded down the hall. Chrissi turned to her sister, who had made her way to the kitchen from where she had been playing with the kids all day. "Thank you, again. Staying for dinner?"

"No, I need to run. Can the kids come to my house tomorrow?" She put her arm around Chrissi's shoulders as she stood at the stove.

"Of course. I can't thank you enough."

"Don't worry about. I love those little kiddos!" She squeezed Chrissi's shoulders and said her goodbyes.

I sat there while they ate, the clatter of forks and the soft thump of little feet swinging beneath the table. Dalton spilled his milk. Chrissi wiped it up without missing a beat. The smells making my mouth water.

After dinner, I watched from the recliner as Chrissi moved from task to task like she was chasing the clock. She scooped up Averi for her bath, toweled her off, then read three books while Dalton begged for four. Finally, one last kiss on a tiny forehead and the kids were asleep.

Then she came to me.

"You ready?" she asked, voice quiet.

I nodded.

She snapped on gloves. Laid out the meds on a fresh towel. Cleaned my port-a-catheter like a pro. Hooked up the line. Checked the feeding tube. Adjusted the wires, the dressings, the edges of the grafts that always pulled just a little too tight when I laid flat.

"Okay," she whispered. "Turn your head."

I did, and she reached for the compression mask. Slipped it over my face, gently pressing it into place, lining up the seams. Her fingers lingered for just a second on my cheek before she stepped back. "Alright, mister. You're good."

She helped me up from the recliner and we walked slowly to the bedroom, Chrissi making sure I didn't step on a stray matchbox car or barbie doll.

I watched her pull back the covers on her side of the bed. She moved slowly now. Finally, still.

The clock said 12:17 a.m.

By the time I woke up to the cereal clinking into bowls and her voice saying, "No, baby, your other shoes," the sun was just peaking over the treetops.

I laid there in the silence that came between socks and zippers and squabbles, thinking about how we were both still in the middle of it.

And she never got to rest.

LET ME BE CLEAR: they don't send you home when you are healed. You go home when the hospital can no longer do anything for you that can't be done at home. I had Integra bandages all over—clear sheets they'd laid across the raw, burned skin. They looked like something out of a butcher's shop. Stuck to every part of my head and upper shoulders. Hurt like hell when they had to be peeled off and replaced, which Chrissi had the pleasure of doing regularly.

Grafted skin sealed my eyes shut before the doctors would cut those tiny pinholes so I could see again six months after the accident. But for months, I was blind. When I could see again, I slept with a blackout mask because I had no eyelids to close over my eyes.

My lips had been burned off too, so they grafted skin over my mouth with the tiniest opening. Couldn't fit anything bigger than a straw through it.

Chrissi, with her crash course on nursing, administered my meds. Kept track of the schedule. Cleaned my wounds. Fed me. Nothing tests a marriage like that.

REBECCA BROUGHT Alison over to see me. Like Averi, she didn't want to even come inside. It had been so long, and she was scared of what she would see. Rebecca had to make her come in. When she did, she screamed until Rebecca had to take her out of the room, like Chrissi had with Averi.

"We will try again soon, Pat, I promise," her stepdad assured me as he followed Rebecca and Alison out of our house.

The fact that my girls, my baby girls, wouldn't even come to me was a whole new torture. I was their dad, and they couldn't tell.

After I had those pinholes and could see a little, I saw Averi run by one day as I was sitting in my recliner. She wouldn't walk by—her fear keeping her uncertain of this creature wearing her dad's clothes. I reached out and grabbed her. Pulled her onto my lap and held her close. At first, she squirmed harder, her nightmares coming true. But I didn't let go until the fear in her body eased and her head dropped to my chest.

"Daddy."

"That's right, baby. It's just Daddy." Her heart finally convincing her mind that it really was me beneath all the bandages.

CHRISTMAS at the firehouse used to be one of my favorite nights of the year. Every December, the station would host a big party—firefighters and their wives—the whole crew. We'd drag in folding tables, string up lights, bring covered dishes and gallons of sweet tea. Loud music, louder laughter. It was something we all looked forward to.

So that year, after I got home from the hospital, I told Chrissi I wanted to go.

"You sure?" she asked, tying a ribbon around a plate of cookies. "We don't have to."

"I'm sure," I said. "I need to."

I got dressed as best I could. Chrissi fixed my collar and buttoned it down for me. We drove to the station in silence, her hand resting on my knee.

When we walked in, conversations trailed off.

"Pat!" one of the guys said, stepping forward. "Good to see you, brother."

I was expecting a hug, but he just patted my shoulder instead—

light, like I might break. Others followed suit. A few handshakes, a couple of quiet "we've been praying for you" comments.

The room was loud. I knew the decorations would fill the walls. There would be tables full of casseroles and cakes. But it didn't feel the same. It wasn't the noise—it was the space. The quiet gaps where I used to be.

I stood there, not knowing what to do with my hands. I tried to join a conversation by the dessert table, but the guys fell silent when I walked up. "Hey, man, you doing all right?" one asked, then the conversation trailed off, no one knowing what to say next.

It was too soon. Things were still too raw. I wasn't just Pat anymore. I was the man who came back from the dead. The one they didn't know how to talk to.

I felt Chrissi come up beside me. "Ready to head out?" she asked.

I nodded. "Yeah. Let's go."

That night, as Chrissi and I were laying in bed, I told her, "It just wasn't the same."

"Pat, I know this has been awful for you, but you don't understand what it was like for everyone else. I felt like you died."

Her statement hung in the air like a gut punch. I couldn't respond. What do you say to that? That there were times I wished I had died?

## 12

## SIDELINES

The sun was already high when I heard the back door slam and the screen bounce once against the frame.

"Daddy! We're gettin' in the pool!" Averi shouted, barefoot and grinning, goggles already halfway up her forehead.

Dalton trailed behind her, dragging a float the size of a small boat. "Mama said it's finally warm enough!"

I stood at the window, watching them run across the deck like it was the best day of their lives. And for them, it probably was.

Chrissi was already outside, spreading towels across the chairs, laughing as she tried to wrestle sunscreen onto our wiggling toddler.

I opened the door just enough to lean out. "Y'all be careful."

Dalton turned around. "You not comin' out, Daddy?"

I hesitated. "Not today, son."

His face fell. "But it's summer! You always get in."

"Yeah," I said. "I know."

I could feel Chrissi's eyes on me from the other side of the pool. She didn't say anything. She just gave me a half smile and went back to rubbing sunscreen on Averi's arms.

The truth was, I couldn't risk it. Couldn't be in the water with them splashing around, not with the trache. One wrong hit, one splash of pool water the wrong way, and it could've landed me back in the hospital. And the skin grafts—they couldn't be in the sun yet. Couldn't risk infection and the breaking down of what had barely started to heal.

Dalton tried again. "What if you just sit by the pool? You don't have to swim."

Chrissi answered before I could. "Let Daddy rest today, kids. He's gotta stay out of the sun for a while."

They didn't argue.

I closed the door gently and went back to the recliner. Turned on the TV, but I couldn't even watch it. Just sat there listening to them laugh outside as the water splashed. Those were the kinds of sounds that used to mean everything was alright. But now, it was just another reminder of something else I couldn't do anymore.

IT HAD BEEN ALMOST a year since the accident when the guys finally talked me into coming back to the firehouse, not for a function, but to visit over coffee like old times. They wanted me back in the house. Said they missed me, and it'd be good for morale.

When I walked through the bay doors, the guys lit up like it was Christmas morning.

"Look who decided to show up!" Neal hollered, coming in for a half hug, half back slap.

"Thought you'd forgotten what a firetruck looked like," another said with a grin.

"Place ain't the same without you," one of the younger guys added.

I smiled, trying to believe them.

The longer I stayed in the firehouse, the more I felt like I could help out again. I did what I could—coiled some hose, checked the gear. But my vision was still shot, and the heat from the truck made my face feel like it was peeling off. Every time I reached for something, someone else rushed in to do it for me.

"You alright?" Neal asked.

"Yeah," I said. "Just hot."

Tones dropped before I could lie any further. House fire. Not far. Everyone scrambled into place. I hesitated, not quite sure what to do.

"You coming?" Chief hollered as he hurried past me to the truck.

I followed out of habit, climbing into the truck like muscle memory could carry me through.

When we got there, I stood back, helmet on, turnout gear half-zipped, trying to find where I fit in.

"Pat—stay close to the truck, alright?" One of them said as they all headed to put out the flames.

I nodded, stepped back.

"Watch your step there," someone else said as I moved to help uncoil some hose.

"Let us handle this part," he added. "You just keep a look out."

I knew what they meant. They were trying to keep me safe. But it didn't feel like safety. It felt like I was in the way. Like they had to babysit me while the house burned.

I watched them go in—tools swinging, commands sharp, fire glowing off their coats. I'd done that a hundred times before. Knew what it felt like to carry the weight, to be needed, to be part of it.

Now I was a liability.

When it was over, we rode back in silence. Nobody said it, but I could feel it—like we all knew something had shifted.

Back at the house, Neal clapped me on the shoulder. "You're always welcome here, man. Always."

I nodded. "Thanks."

I didn't go back.

## 13

## DENIAL

For the next few years, I would have surgery after surgery. Fixing this issue or that one, moving skin and taking it away, attaching and reattaching pieces until I felt like a patchwork quilt. I had about one surgery a month for years. And the surgeries were seldom outpatient. I would go up and spend a week in the hospital, come home and recover for three weeks, then go again for the next round. They used the skin on my thighs to replace the melted skin on my head. They fashioned eyelids from flaps of skin, but I still couldn't blink or close my eyes. I would have to pinch the skin closed over my eyes at night to sleep. But that was better than having to put bandages over them to block out the light. Not that I really wanted to sleep. Sleep meant returning to the nightmarish fire that caused this hell.

They put magnetic implants on the sides of my head so that prosthetic ears could be attached. They turned the skin around my mouth inside out to fashion what passed as my mouth. This allowed them to take out the feeding tube and let me eat again.

They tried to make me look and function as normal as possible. But that was still far from enough. The fire didn't just take my face—it took everything that made my life feel normal. My confidence. My career. My comfort. After the fire, everything took effort. And when I did make the effort, it was seldom worth it. I basically stayed at my house. I couldn't drive. I didn't really want to see anyone. Not because I didn't want the company—I didn't want the stares or the pity. My close friends and family were the only ones I wanted around because they wouldn't stare or coddle me. If anybody wanted to see me, they had to come to my house. Not many did. And I didn't blame them.

FROM THE TIME of the accident, my recovery became both mine and Chrissi's full-time job. First, it was round the clock with no holidays. Then slowly, it shifted to being just your normal 40 hours a week, plus lots of overtime. Yet this job came with bills instead of a paycheck. There was no way for either of us to earn money. We had to rely on the insurance money to keep us afloat. Dad, Bill, and Travis did their best to keep the store running so that we could have something coming in, but it wasn't long before Dad decided to sell the store. Bill was frustrated, and Travis was out of a job. And Chrissi and I were running out of money.

We began selling things to pay the bills. Little things at first that we knew would make quick cash—things like my guns and tools. Then the bigger things that brought larger paydays. The boat went, then the four-wheelers. Traded the cars in to buy a little cheap truck that was just enough to get us around. Finally, after two years of trying to hold everything together, we had to surrender to something I dreaded doing–selling our dream home.

When Chrissi first got pregnant with Dalton, her parents had built a large room onto the front of their house, attached to Chrissi's old room. It had its own entrance, but no bathroom. It was like a little studio apartment. We moved in there, us and three kids sharing this tiny little space and the single bathroom in the main house. We were so cramped, and emotions and tempers were high, but having her parents around to help with the kids was a huge blessing. We would talk and dream of building a house so big that we wouldn't even see each other pass in the halls. I couldn't wait to make that happen, but I knew that meant I had to get well enough to get back to work.

I HADN'T LISTENED to the doctors when they told me so many things would be different. I hadn't wanted to hear the truth. I had ignored it and shoved it down and refused to look in the mirror at what was actually happening to me.

I still wasn't looking, but maybe just maybe, if I put my head down long enough, kept going long enough, just like Chrissi had for months in the hospital and then the past few years at home, we would come out of this. We had built it all once; we could build it again. I looked different, but I was still strong, fit, and had my mind. The medication helped me to keep functioning. It kept the pain at bay. I could learn to ignore the stares, the fear in people's eyes, especially kids, when they saw me. I could get us back to where we were before. All I thought about was getting back to that point, that moment. Before.

I'D SPENT ALL those days in the hospital with a steady drip of every painkiller known to man running through my veins. Then, when I first went home from the hospital, the medications went through the port-a-cath, those little suction tubes that Chrissi had to administer. Eventually, the feeding tube came out, and I was able to swallow. That meant the medications changed to your typical pain pills. They sent me home with a prescription for twenty-four pills, meant to last an entire month. That was it, less than one a day for a month. So, I took those pills and called them back a little over a week later and asked for more, which they gave me, without any questions asked. Anyone seeing my history could not imagine how bad the pain was, and happily prescribed whatever they thought might make it more manageable.

But I was not taking the pills as prescribed. I took them as I thought I needed. Every few hours, sometimes more than one at a time. Because if one worked, two were better. It wasn't only the physical pain that I was trying to avoid. I couldn't face the loss of my business, our home, or...possibly our future.

Chrissi noticed me taking more pills than usual. But she couldn't say anything to me about it. She didn't know what I was going through.

"Bill, I can't find him!" Chrissi's voice shook on the other end of the line.

"Well he couldn't have gone far. How long since you saw him?" Bill asked. But this wasn't the first time they had this conversation.

"It's been hours, Bill. I can't just leave the kids and go look for him!"

"I know, I know. I'm on my way. Don't worry, Chrissi. I'll find him."

I heard the crunch of the leaves and footsteps coming up behind me. I didn't move, as if whoever had been sent out this time to find me wouldn't be able to see me sitting here on the ground, leaned up against the rough bark at the base of the oak tree.

"Hey, man." Bill sat down next to me, staring off into space like I was. "Chrissi's worried you know. Says it's been hours this time."

"Yep."

He opened his mouth as if he were about to say something but then stopped. Instead, he let out a sigh and continued to sit by my side, staring with me into the captivating nothing straight ahead without saying a word. *He read me well.* I saw him take out his phone and type something, then slip it back in his pocket. Probably an "I found him," text to Chrissi.

Wasn't sure how much time passed, but it was enough that the sky darkened, and the air grew colder. "You hungry?" he asked.

I turned my head, finally making eye contact with him after all of that time. "I could eat," I responded.

Bill then got up and extended his hand toward me. I waved him off, planting my hands on the ground and pushing myself up. As I did, my hunting jacket rose up on my side, uncovering the pistol I had tucked into my waistband. *Did he see it? He had to.* Bill took a step back and looked at me and paused. *Here it comes. A lecture about how much everybody cares about me,* I thought. He finally said something. "How about some pulled pork with baked beans and slaw?" We smiled at each other.

"There's nothing like it," I said.

He nodded in agreement. "Yeah, life wouldn't be the same without it."

I felt his eyes piercing through my heart. "That thing's been going strong on the menu for years. It ain't going nowhere anytime soon," I said.

He smiled, then responded. "Good."

# 14

# EXPOSED

One day I'd be okay. The next, not so much. I didn't know how to deal with my reality—so I ran from it. Hid in the woods. Hid behind jokes. Hid behind sunglasses.

It had been one of those days. The kind where everything gets on your nerves. The kids were loud, and the little apartment felt like it was getting even smaller by the hour. Between the toys in every corner and the daily arguments, there wasn't any room for peace.

I was sitting on the edge of the bed, trying to get a break from the noise, when Chrissi came in and shut the door behind her. She didn't say anything at first. Just looked at me like she was trying to read my mind. Then she sat down beside me. "We need to get outta here."

I looked over at her. "Don't you think I want to? That's all I am trying to do!"

"No, Pat," she took a long breath, as if having this argument again for the five hundredth time was the last thing she wanted. "I mean, away. Just for a few days. The guys are planning a weekend down at Sardis for the Fourth. Campers, tents, barbecue, the whole deal. Just like we used to. Everybody's bringing their kids. They want us to come."

I didn't say anything. Just stared at the wall for a second, thinking about everything I couldn't do. Couldn't swim, couldn't be out in the sun.

Chrissi nudged my knee. "Pat. You need this. We all do."

I let out a breath. I was tired of being in the way, tired of being looked at, tired of saying no. And she was right—we needed to get away. Even if it was just for a weekend.

"Alright," I said. "Let's go camping."

We set up the tents and began grilling the steaks. It felt like old times again. Until I saw *her*. This little girl from the site next to us kept watching me. I could tell she wanted to play with my girls, but every time she saw me, she froze. She appeared to be studying me, with this look of half horror and half curiosity on her face. I didn't blame her. I looked like something out of a nightmare.

Yet each time I looked over, she was a little closer. A little braver, but still obviously scared.

So, I met her halfway. "Y'all seen that big ol' lion out in the woods?" I shouted. "It got me last summer! Took my ears and everything!" Kids screamed and scattered.

Except her. She marched up and said, "There's not really a lion, is there?"

I leaned in. "Oh yeah. Gotta be careful out here."

She squinted and then smiled. After that, she ran off with the rest of 'em and began playing with my girls.

I loved that I could make her smile and erase her fear. I wish I could erase mine. I was still the same guy I had been a few years before—an outgoing jokester wanting to hang out with my friends and have fun. But people didn't see that Pat. They saw the scars the burns left behind. They saw a face that had no ears or nose. The face with no lips or eyelids. They probably saw a monster. But I wasn't one; I was just Pat.

It was becoming more evident that the "before" was a distant memory of a time that I could never get back to, and the "after" just plain sucked. I walked back to our tent, found my medication, and tossed back a few pills to numb my spiraling thoughts.

. . .

My vision improved enough that I could begin driving again. I even started driving myself to doctor's appointments to give Chrissi a break from at least one of her burdens. To me, it was a small victory in the midst of all the losses that had been piling up one after the other for nearly two years.

I was out running errands in my little truck. Next stop—the bank drive-thru. Not thinking about the compression stocking cap on my head that had replaced the bandages, I pulled up.

"I need to deposit these checks," I told the teller.

"Ju...Just...a second," she stammered.

I sat there waiting, drumming my fingers on the steering wheel to the music in my truck.

Suddenly, I saw cops pull up with full lights and sirens. I started looking around, trying to figure out what on earth was going on.

Next thing I know, I've got police officers with guns drawn, pointed at me! "Put your hands on the steering wheel! Keep your hands where I can see 'em," the officer screamed.

"What? I'm just making a deposit, not trying to rob the place," I joked. Then I realized that was exactly what they thought I was doing.

"Guys, relax, it's me. Pat."

One stepped closer, looking fully into the cab. "Pat! What on earth! The teller said there was a masked gunman out here!"

I laughed with them, but inside I wanted to scream. Turns out the young teller hit the silent alarm. The bank had been robbed just a couple of weeks before, so nerves were high. She panicked. I can't blame her.

They apologized once they realized who I was. The bank president himself even called me. I told him it was alright. What else could I say? Wasn't their fault that some guy in what looked like a ski mask scared the teller. I wasn't trying to. I was just trying to help Chrissi.

Just when I started to gain traction with adjusting to my new reality, I was reminded that as much as I might try to convince myself and others differently, I wasn't the old Pat anymore. It was a constant ebb and flow of promises, followed by pain. Making people laugh and overcome their fears seemed to promise that the old Pat was coming back. But then, causing fear and panic brought the pain of knowing that what's gone can never be recovered. Just ups and downs, with more of the negative. Funny how the downs are easier to maintain, following a slow and steady descent towards rock bottom.

People talk about hitting rock bottom like it's one clean moment. Like it is one hard hit and then you can start climbing out. The truth is, there are rocks on the way down that you bounce off of as you fall. Protruding ones that leave bruises you don't always see until later. Sharp, jagged ones that leave cuts that fester. Those rocks are the friends that stop calling. The client who quietly pulls their business without ever saying why. The small humiliations you don't talk about.

I didn't like where I was headed, but I felt that there was nothing I could do about it. Glancing at my truck, I realized at least I can still drive. I left with no intention of coming back. I climbed into the cab of that truck, pointed it north, and drove. No plan. No goodbye. Just a man with little eyesight and a whole lot of pain.

I ended up hours north, in the mountains of Tennessee. Parked under the trees. Pistol under the seat. I let the silence do the talking. *Maybe that was a mistake.* I started thinking about the psychiatrist I was seeing. Talk therapy. More meds. He'd sit there across from me in that chair, nodding and scribbling, but nothing he said ever fixed what was broken in me. No counselor can bring back the man I once was, and no pill in this world can give me back my face. I tried numbing the pain and burying it, but it didn't go away. I realized that if I don't face this head-on, I would be running from it the rest of my life. *I ain't a runner. That's not Pat Hardison.*

Realizing I had to make a choice, a line from *Shawshank Redemption* floated through my mind: "Get busy living or get busy dying." And just like that, I saw my kids.

Dalton swinging a bat. Alison chasing Averi through the sprinkler. Sticky hands. Skinned knees. And I knew I couldn't leave them.

That revelation didn't heal me, but it was God's extended hand out of the pit. I was still breathing. And if I'm breathing, it can only mean one thing—that God wasn't done with me. I packed up the pity party and turned the truck back towards Mississippi. Once I got back home, I got busy living.

# 15

# HOPE

Before we even moved out of our dream house, God showed us that there was still hope ahead. We were standing in the kitchen when she told me. I'd just come in from the shop, and she was holding that little plastic stick like it might bite her. She didn't even say anything at first. Just held it out toward me, wide-eyed.

I looked at the two pink lines and raised my eyebrows. "Well...I guess that's clear."

She laughed—nervous, tired, hopeful. "Guess so."

It wasn't planned. But it didn't matter. I walked over, wrapped my arms around her, and whispered, "Maybe this is God tellin' us we're gonna make it after all."

A few months later, we were sitting in that dim ultrasound room, watching the screen light up with the image of a tiny human. Then the tech said, "Looks like you're having a boy," and I felt something loosen in my chest that I didn't know I'd been holding.

A boy. Our second son. Braden.

I stared at that grainy printout for a long time when we got home. Held it in my hand like it was a promise. A new baby. Maybe even a new me. I thought, *maybe this is God's way of showing me things are finally turning around*. A second chance to get it right.

Braden came into this world ready to go. And then—almost before we caught our breath—God added another blessing. Cullen. Another boy. Another round of sleepless nights, little socks, and tiny fists around my fingers.

The thing about those two boys is—they never knew me before.

To them, I had always looked this way. The face with no ears. The skin pulled tight. The voice a little strained. The prosthetics. The pills on the counter. The naps I had to take in the middle of the day. That was just Dad.

They didn't flinch. Didn't stare. They climbed up in my lap like it was the safest place in the world. I'd feel their little hands touch my face and ask questions like, "Does it hurt today, Daddy?"

They never knew what I'd lost. They just knew they were loved.

And they loved me right back. As broken and patched together as I was.

That love—pure, unfiltered, unconditional—it did something to me. I don't think they'll ever fully understand how much it helped. How much they helped. Because in a world that felt like it didn't recognize me anymore, they did.

They saw Dad.

And sometimes, that was enough to keep me going.

I FOCUSED on getting back to work. With some help, I opened another tire shop in town with a new business partner. Was even able to hire Travis back. It didn't take long for Travis and me to find our old rhythm and return to selling tires and wheels like they were water in a desert. The first year, we did $1.4 million in sales. We were beginning to turn things around. Pay bills. The conversations about that new house changed from arguments about what we didn't have to a real possibility of what we might have again.

Opening the new tire store felt like a fresh start. Business was steady, and for the first time in a long time, I felt like I was building something again instead of just surviving.

. . .

RIDING on the high of new babies and a new business, Chrissi and I did something we hadn't dared to do in years—we dreamed big.

We bought land out in a subdivision called Bartlett Woods. A beautiful lot with space to breathe, tucked back far enough to feel private but still close enough to town. It felt like a stake in the ground. Like we were saying, we made it through the fire, and we're not just surviving anymore—we're building.

We'd talk through plans late at night, her legs curled under her on the couch, me stretched out with a notebook in my lap. She had ideas for the kitchen—big island, cabinets, open shelves. I wanted a garage big enough to park a boat and still have room to tinker. We both agreed: we were going to have space. No more tripping over toys, no more bumping into each other in tight hallways. We'd shared that tiny apartment at her mama's house for too long. It was time.

The house wasn't as massive as we used to joke about when we were crammed into one room with three kids—even so, with over 6,500 square feet of floor space, it felt enormous. Almost too good to be true.

We designed it with intention. Not just to live in—but to build equity. The plan was to finish it, live there for a bit, then sell it and roll the profit into the next one. Maybe keep doing that. Build. Sell. Build again. It was smart. It was solid. And for the first time in forever, we weren't just catching up—we were getting ahead.

I'd walk through the framing with Dalton and Braden in tow, their feet crunching sawdust, pointing out where their rooms would be.

"This one's yours, Bubba," I told Braden once, lifting him up so he could see out the window. "You'll be able to watch deer from here come winter."

Dalton grinned, wide-eyed and gap-toothed. "Can we put a trampoline in the backyard?"

I ruffled his hair. "We'll see."

Chrissi stood across the room, her hand tracing where the kitchen counter would go. Sunlight poured through the empty window frames, lighting her up like she was already home.

And in that moment, I wasn't thinking about my scars. Neither was I thinking about the pills or the pain.

I was thinking about drywall and paint colors. About dinners at a big kitchen table with five kids. About rebuilding a life that didn't just work—but one we were proud of.

I'd carried debt and shame for so long, I couldn't remember what it felt like to breathe easy. I wasn't about to go back there. This house was our chance to do it differently. To do it better. For the kids and for us.

For once, the future didn't feel like a burden. It felt like a blueprint.

I STARTED COACHING Little League baseball, something I'd always dreamed of doing. I'd played on those same fields as a kid, and there was something special about coming full circle—sharing my favorite sport with my son and helping shape a team of eager little players who still believed they might be the next big MLB star. We picked the team's name, set the first practice, rounded up the gear, and headed to the field. I threw on my baseball cap and dark sunglasses—something I'd always worn, but now they felt more like armor than shade—and tried to shake the nerves as we walked toward the dugout.

"Hey everyone, I'm Coach Pat. Y'all excited to play ball?" I asked with a grin, but the excitement I felt didn't bounce back. The kids stood still, uncertain. I saw the fear in their eyes—that same flicker I'd seen too many times before. So, I went ahead and called it out. "I think y'all are wondering about my face." A few timid nods confirmed it. "I know, it looks kinda scary. But it's just skin. I was a firefighter, and I got hurt in a fire. Y'all know what firefighters do, right?" More nods this time, the tension easing. "Well, when I was putting out a fire, I got burned. That's all. Nothing to be scared of. Now let's play ball, okay?" I could tell they were still unsure, so I pulled off one of my prosthetic ears and held it toward them. "I can't hear you. I said—OK?" That broke the tension.

They giggled, some pointing, others covering their mouths, and shouted back, "OK!"

I clapped my hands. "Great! Now let's grab our gloves and get on the field." And just like that, most of them did.

Except for one little boy. His face crumpled, and he ran to his mom, tears already falling. I walked toward them slowly, trying not to make it worse.

"I'm so sorry, Pat," she said as she held him close. "He's just... scared."

I nodded. "I get it." But the closer I got, the harder he cried, so I stopped. I'd heard those cries before with my own kids in the early days, when they didn't quite understand who I was anymore. But the difference was, I could pick them up. I could hold them tight until they remembered my arms were still Dad's arms, even if my face didn't look like Dad's face. That doesn't work with a stranger's kid. I looked at the mom and said gently, "I'm happy to help him find another team if you'd like."

She looked down at her son, clinging to her, his face buried in her stomach. Her mouth opened like she might say something, but then she just nodded—quick and tight—like she didn't want to make a scene. She gave me a small, apologetic smile, the kind people give when they wish things were different but don't know how to fix them. Her eyes flicked around the field, then back to her son. She nodded again, fuller this time, as if accepting the situation, turned and led him toward the parking lot, her hand rubbing circles on his back.

I watched them go, wishing I could've made it easier for both of them, but knowing I couldn't.

I turned back to the field, where the other kids were already tossing balls and chasing each other like nothing had happened. I adjusted my sunglasses and called out to the team, grateful the glasses were dark enough to hide the tears.

## 16

## DEPENDENT

Pain was still an everyday, all day, thing, physically and mentally. And all I wanted to do was numb that pain.

I had been on pain pills for a long time. Lots of them. It started with pain medication for the daily procedures and constant surgeries required to keep me healing. Though they wouldn't prescribe a large script, it was nothing for me to call a few days later and get it renewed.

"Yeah, the prescription was for 24 pills. I took one about every six hours this week, so I'm out already, and wondered if you could call in a refill?"

"Sure thing Mr. Hardison, I will get that sent right over to your pharmacy."

It wasn't just one doctor prescribing them, either. I had appointments with surgeons, psychiatrists, physical therapists, you name it. And they would each give me a prescription. Back then, it was easy to get pain pills. Too easy. They didn't have the systems they've got now. No one was tracking it. No red flags. No questions asked. When I told them I had taken one every six hours, they would believe me. They had no idea it was more like three pills every four hours, and the prescription from their office had run out days before.

And no one ever said, "Pat, you need pain management." Not once. So, I managed it myself.

BY THE TIME I was home from the burn unit, I was already dependent. I just didn't know what it was at the time. All I knew was that when I ran out, I got sick. Shaking. Cold sweats. Every muscle aching like I was still in the burn unit. And about the time I would think, *I can't keep doing this*, I would have another surgery—more pain, more legitimate prescriptions.

Eventually, one doctor mentioned a pain specialist.

"Mr. Hardison, I think it's time we get someone to help manage this long-term."

I nodded like it was news to me, like I hadn't been barely holding on for months. "Yeah. That'd be good."

I showed up to the clinic a week later, slouched in the vinyl seat while Chrissi filled out the paperwork. She glanced over at me once, pen still moving. "You gonna be honest with him?"

I didn't answer.

The waiting room was full of people like me. Limping. Pale. Worn out. Some didn't look hurt at all—just tired in a different way. I didn't meet their eyes. Maybe it was because I didn't want to see myself in them.

When the nurse called me back, I followed her into a small room that smelled like alcohol wipes and cheap leather. The specialist walked in a few minutes later—middle-aged, glasses hanging low on his nose, clipboard in hand.

"Mr. Hardison," he said, flipping through my chart. "Looks like you've had quite a journey."

"That's one way to put it."

He didn't laugh. Just kept reading.

"Your med list is...," he paused, raised an eyebrow, "impressive."

"So is the pain," I said.

That earned a smile. "Fair enough."

He asked questions. Lots of them. Type of pain. Location. Triggers. How much sleep I was getting. How many pills I took and when. I told him what he wanted to hear.

He tapped his pen against the clipboard, thinking. "Alright. You've got unmanaged chronic pain layered over acute trauma. We're going to streamline this. One medication, steady dose, closely monitored. I also want you checking in every month."

I nodded, relieved. For once, someone wasn't just scribbling out a script and sending me on my way.

He handed me the paper. "This is long-acting. Should help with the peaks and valleys."

He didn't understand how grateful I was. *Finally, I'm going to get fixed,* I thought. That first night, I took the pill exactly how he told me. No extra. No skipping. No chasing the edge of pain like it was a moving target. And for the first time in weeks, I slept. The next morning, the pain wasn't gone. But it wasn't screaming either. Just a dull throb I could walk around with.

For a little while, it helped. I followed the schedule. Took the right dose. Even brought the bottle to appointments like I was proving something.

But the pain never let up. Not really.

It crouched in the corners of my day, waiting. Reminding me it was still there. Still mine.

And before long, I started filling in the gaps again. One pill became two. Or three when the weather turned. I told myself it was just temporary. Just until things eased up. But things didn't ease up.

ONE DAY I was curled up on the couch, miserable. Dad stood over me, watching me rock back and forth, soaked in sweat.

"I can't stand this," he said. "I'm going to find you something."

He came back a few hours later with a fresh supply of pills. I didn't ask where he got them. I could think of a few options. Owning a tire store, we had our share of customers who came in wanting to buy fancy rims with a handful of cash. Guess it was a full-circle type situation where Dad had become a customer of theirs. I didn't care either way. The pills took away how terrible I felt, so I didn't say a word to him, except…"thank you." The next time I ran out of pills, I just let Dad know, and he took care of it again.

Dad didn't bring me the gun when I begged for it. But he brought me those pills. That was his way of helping. I didn't judge him for it.

And somewhere along the line, he started keeping some for himself. "I gave you what I could get," he said one time, handing me twenty pills when I'd asked for thirty.

I knew but I didn't say anything. We were circling the same drain.

Mom stayed quiet. She always had. Old-school kind of woman that obeyed her husband and didn't make waves. I wish she'd said something, raised hell, slammed a door. Maybe it would've made a difference. But honestly? We probably wouldn't have listened.

## 17

# ADDICTION

I stood at the kitchen sink, coffee in one hand, three pills in the other. Dry-swallowed 'em without thinking. No water. No hesitation. Just part of the routine. I'd already taken two earlier, but the pain was back—and with it, the shakes. So, I did what I had to. I took three more.

Chrissi walked through the kitchen just as I shoved the bottle back into the drawer.

She didn't say anything. Didn't have to. She saw. I knew she did. But neither of us wanted to deal with what it meant, so we did what we always did—we kept moving.

TAKING that many pills didn't get me high. It didn't even give me a buzz. I had built up such a tolerance; it didn't matter if I took one or four. The only difference was whether I could make it through the next few hours without getting sick. I wasn't chasing a high. I was trying to stay level. Trying not to throw up or curl up in a ball on the bathroom floor.

. . .

THAT'S the trap of opioid addiction. It starts in a hospital bed. With real pain. Real doctors. Real prescriptions. So, you think it's safe. You think it's different.

You think *you're* different.

But before long, you're doing things you swore you'd never do—lying, hiding, justifying your actions to make it through the day. You tell yourself you're managing it. But really, it's managing you.

And somewhere along the way, it becomes easier to hate yourself than to stop. Looking in the mirror was still hard. Still the same burned face. Still, the missing ears. But now it wasn't just what I looked like that was hard to see—it was what I'd become.

AT ONE POINT, I could make the pills from doctors last two, or maybe even three weeks. The rest? I bought. Whether it was strangers or friends, it didn't matter. I didn't have to go far. Everybody knew somebody. And most folks didn't ask questions. They just named their price.

Addiction doesn't take a day off. Doesn't care if it's Christmas morning or your kid's birthday or the day you swore you were done. When you're in it, you're in it.

I never called myself an addict. Addicted...maybe. But not an addict. Addicts were weak. Out of control. I was still making payroll. Still changing diapers. Still smiling at church. Addicts were homeless and jobless. Held signs at intersections. They'd lost everything. I still had a house. I still owned a business. Still showed up to coach my son's Little League team. I was paying bills and making dinner plans.

But I was lying.

I WAS JUST as hooked as anybody out there.

That's what makes opioid addiction so dangerous. It hides behind the doctor's notes and surgery scars and real pain. You start from something that makes sense. Something that hurts. And when the hurting doesn't stop, you tell yourself you deserve relief. You've earned it. It's just one more pill. Just for today. Until one day becomes every day.

We like to draw lines in our minds—between "those people" and "us." But addiction doesn't care about lines. It doesn't care if you wear a badge or own a business or sing in the church choir. It'll hide behind all of those different faces just the same.

And the worst part is—you still think you're in control.

THING IS, this wasn't just me. It wasn't rare. This was happening all over the country. Starting in the '90s, drug companies started pushing pain meds like they were candy. OxyContin hit the shelves, and doctors were told pain was the "fifth vital sign." They had to treat it. Fix it. So they handed out prescriptions like Tic Tacs.

Between 1999 and 2010, opioid sales in the U.S. quadrupled. Overdose deaths more than doubled.[1] In 2010 alone, enough pills were prescribed to keep every adult in America medicated 24 hours a day for a full month.

That's how bad it got.

And a lot of those pills didn't come from drug dealers. They came from people like me. Like you. Nurses. Police officers. Grandmas on Social Security. Folks who needed cash more than medication.

Some gave me their pills out of pity. They saw the scars, the eyes, the face. They wanted to help. Others were just making rent. A bottle of pills could go for hundreds. And when you're broke, tired, and forgotten by the system, that math starts to make sense.

That's how broken it all was.

You could walk into a doctor's office with a backache and leave with a bottle that might ruin your life. One script. One refill. That's all it took. Those meds—they didn't care if you were careful. They didn't care what kind of person you were before. They rewire your brain. Trick it. Make you believe you need them. And then—you do.

---

1. https://www.congress.gov/crs-product/IF12260#:~:text=Between%201999%20and%202010%2C%20theof%20the%20recent%20opioid%20crisis

Not to feel good. Just to function and not be sick.

Because when you stop—just for a day—the withdrawal comes.

And there I was, an ex-firefighter who was just another statistic—trying to survive in my personalized, living hell.

# 18

# LOSS

I remember standing at the counter one afternoon at the shop, counting out two hundred dollars like it was nothing. Two crisp hundreds, gone in seconds. Just to make it to the next day. That kind of spending adds up fast. Six grand a month for years. That's somebody's salary. Three, four years of that kind of spending, and it adds up to more than just money lost. It costs you everything. Unless you've got millions coming in, you are spending the money that should be for the mortgage, the insurance, and the groceries.

After I opened the new shop and could start providing again, Chrissi and I would have a system where the bills were sent to the shop and she would trust me to take care of them. I did. For a while. Until my "pain management" became more of a priority. Those bills weren't always getting paid. But since the bills kept coming to the shop, she never saw the late notices or the final warnings. She assumed I was taking care of them, just like before, and I was happy to go along with it.

. . .

CHRISSI ALSO KNEW I wasn't taking my meds as prescribed, and she knew Dad had his way of adding to the number of pills I had available, but she didn't truly know the depth of how many and how often. No one did. I kept the pills stashed where people, especially Chrissi and the kids, wouldn't find them. She didn't ask too many questions, and I certainly didn't give her too many answers. She was finally coming out from the fire hose of suffering that had been holding her down and threatening to drown her. Other than expressing her concerns about some of my dad's acquaintances being around the kids, she didn't say much. I guess she was just so grateful for some of the weight to be lifted.

BUT NOT EVERYONE STAYED QUIET. One day at the shop, Travis noticed that I slipped a guy some money in exchange for a small folded up Ziplock. I stuck it in my pocket and headed back to my office, unaware of the witness.

He waited until the next day to say something. "Hey, Pat, I need to talk to you for a second. I saw what happened yesterday, it looked like you bought some pills. That's not okay, man. If you need some help, I can get you some help. Get you off those things."

"You work for me. You do what I tell you and don't ask questions about this kind of stuff," I told him.

After that, Travis decided he couldn't work for me anymore. I watched him walk out the door. Part of me wanted to call him back. Apologize. Say he was right. But the louder part—the addict part—just muttered, "His loss."

That's how addiction communicates. It always has the last word.

WE WERE BUILDING our big house out at Bartlett Woods, using a construction loan for about $200,000. As we moved the construction loan over to a mortgage, the house appraised for closer to $500K. We were thrilled! The plan was in action. Now all we had to do was sell it before the first mortgage payment, and we would be sitting on a profit of $300K—enough to build it all over again, out of our own pockets.

It had been four years since my accident, and I thought we were finally pulling ahead. The shop was bringing in money, the house was coming together, and the kids were healthy. For the first time since the fire, I felt like maybe—just maybe—we'd made it through the worst of it.

Then the bottom fell out.

It started slowly. A customer here or there who said they'd come back next paycheck—and didn't. Then bigger jobs that used to be easy sells started falling through. I'd call folks to follow up, and they'd say, "Man, I just can't swing it right now." Over and over again. Couldn't get credit. Couldn't get approved. Couldn't even get a call back from their bank.

That's when I started hearing the words "housing crisis" on the news. "Market correction." "Subprime loans." Sounded like a bunch of Wall Street nonsense at first. But I saw it clearly enough on my end. Folks were losing their houses left and right. Foreclosures popped up like dandelions. House prices dropped like they were made of paper. You'd see a house listed for $400K one month, and by the next it was down to $275K—and still no buyers.

People who'd bought during the boom were underwater, owing more than their place was worth. Couldn't refinance. Couldn't sell. They couldn't even get out from under it if they wanted to. And the banks? They slammed the doors shut. No more loans. No more second chances. Just silence. I remember thinking, *How does everything change this fast?*

Folks stopped buying tires unless they were bald and steel was showing. We'd gone from selling chrome wheels and lift kits to barely getting people in the door. Money got tight. Then tighter. Then impossible.

We were holding all this debt—on the house, the business, everything. And suddenly, it didn't matter how hard we worked. We couldn't dig out of it.

The dream we'd built—6500 square feet of hope and second

chances—started feeling like a weight around my neck. The walls got closer. The payments got heavier. The future we'd been building toward just...cracked.

That's what nobody tells you about these big economic crashes. They say it's about interest rates or stock indexes. But down here on the ground, it's your marriage. Your business. Your livelihood. It's staring at a checkbook with no answers and no backup. It's watching everything you fought for get stripped away and realizing you can't stop it.

In one short year we went from believing things had turned around, to scrambling every month for survival. And the pressure never let up. Not once.

WHEN THE MORTGAGE became something I couldn't pay, I didn't mention it. I just pushed to sell the house. But because the economy was so bad, our hope of selling it for $500K was out the window. I kept lowering the price, but there were no takers. I couldn't sell it fast enough to get out from under the mortgage.

I was at the shop when my phone buzzed in my pocket. I didn't answer right away. Figured it could wait. But it buzzed again. And again. By the third time, I wiped my hands on a rag and pulled it out.

It was Chrissi.

I answered. "Hey, what's going on?"

Her voice was shaking. "Some man just walked up to the backyard and handed me an eviction notice!"

"What?"

"An eviction notice! He said my name, asked if I was Mrs. Hardison, then handed it to me and left. Just like that."

I was already heading back to my office. "What does it say?"

She was quiet for a second. Then I heard her voice crack. "It says we're being foreclosed on, Pat. We have thirty days to move out."

The words hit like a punch. I looked down at the oil and dust covering my boots. My whole body went hot.

"Thirty days," she repeated. "And anything we leave behind becomes property of the bank."

I swallowed hard. "Okay, okay. It's probably a mistake. I'll call the bank. I'll get it straightened out."

She didn't answer right away.

"Chrissi," I said again, softer this time, "I'll handle it. Don't worry."

But I could hear the edge in her voice when she finally spoke. "Is it a mistake, Pat?"

I opened my mouth to lie. To say something comforting. But nothing came out.

There wasn't a mistake. There weren't any misplaced checks or clerical errors. Just a drawer in my office full of unopened bills. Envelopes stacked beside an orange prescription bottle I kept refilling instead of facing the truth.

"No," I finally admitted. "It's not."

Silence on the other end. I could hear the kids laughing in the background, playing like their whole world wasn't about to change... again.

Chrissi's voice dropped. "You should've told me."

"I know," I said. "I just...I thought I could fix it. Thought the house would sell."

I stood there in the middle of the shop, surrounded by tires, oil stains, and a thousand busted dreams. I realized that I couldn't even fix the damage I'd already done.

CHRISSI DIDN'T WAIT. As soon as she hung up the phone, she started grabbing boxes—whatever she could find. Old moving tubs from the garage. Plastic bins. Trash bags. Anything with room to shove our life into.

By the time I got home, the living room looked like a war zone. Toys scattered, clothes half-folded, kitchen stuff dumped into open bins.

"We've got thirty days, Pat," she said without looking up, her hands moving fast. "We are not leaving our stuff behind for them."

I stood in the doorway, guilt sticking to me like sweat. "We'll figure it out," I said.

She slammed a cabinet door. "They're gonna auction it off, Pat. People are already circling, waiting to snatch it up for pennies."

She was right. We'd tried listing it. Set the price at appraisal. Dropped it lower. Still no bites. Why would they pay full price when they could wait and get it for a third of that? All they had to do was let the clock run out.

A few days later, I pulled into the driveway and saw a truck from the gas company parked out front. A guy with work gloves was kneeling by the propane tank, unhooking the lines.

"Hey," I called, walking over. "What's going on?"

"Order came in to collect the tank," he said, not looking at me. "And the logs inside."

He went back inside and returned with the gas logs from our fireplace, rocks and all. Had scraped them up and put them in a bag. Hauled it all away like he was taking out the trash.

Chrissi had to start cooking on a hot plate we plugged in on the kitchen counter. The gas stove was useless now—just another reminder of what we'd lost.

We started selling everything that wasn't nailed down. And some things that were. The theater room upstairs, with those big reclining chairs and surround sound? Gone. Some guy from two towns over came with a trailer, handed us cash, and hauled it all off like it meant nothing.

Every sale felt like a little more of our life slipping away. I kept trying to tell Chrissi—and myself—that we'd come back from this. That if we could just sell enough, scrape enough together, maybe the bank would stop the process.

"We're gonna catch up," I said more than once.

But she didn't say anything anymore when I said stuff like that. Just kept packing.

And as the deadline crept closer, I stopped saying it too. Truth was, there wasn't enough to sell. Not even close. We were losing the house. And this time, I couldn't pretend otherwise.

CHRISSI WAS PACKING up our bedroom closet, working her way through the shelves and the boxes I hadn't touched in years. She reached for my old fire gear, the turnout pants still stiff from time and memory, and tossed them into the pile for donation.

That's when she found the bottle.

I heard her voice from inside the closet. Not loud. Just sharp. "Pat?"

I didn't answer right away. I already knew what she'd found.

She stepped out into the room, holding up the orange bottle like the proof it was. "This was in your boot," she said. "Why would you put this in your boot?"

I tried to play dumb. "I don't know. Probably forgot it was in there."

She stared at me. "You forgot a full bottle of oxycodone was in your boot?"

I shrugged. "It's old."

That's when she dropped the other one. That one was pulled from the pocket of an old hunting jacket. She picked it up. "This one old too?"

I sat on the edge of the bed, hands in my lap, staring at the floor.

She kept digging. Fire department duffel. Bottom drawer. A pair of sneakers I hadn't worn in years.

Each one held a piece of the truth I'd been hiding—and a piece of the marriage she thought she still had.

She didn't yell. She didn't scream. That might've been easier.

She just sat down across from me on the edge of the bed and whispered, "Pat, you've got to get help."

I shook my head slow. "I'm not like that. I'm not some junkie."

"You are addicted to these pills" she said, tears welling in her eyes. "You just don't want to admit it."

"I need it," I snapped. "You don't understand the pain. You don't know what it's like to wake up and already feel like you're burning alive. I'm not using for fun, Chrissi. I'm surviving."

She wiped at her face, hands trembling. "No, you're not. You're disappearing. One pill at a time."

She begged me. Pleaded. But in that moment, I still believed the lie that had taken root years before—that I couldn't make it through the day without the pills.

It wasn't long after that I brought up moving in with my parents.

"No," she said flatly. "Absolutely not."

"It's just temporary," I tried. "We could save some money, figure things out."

"Your dad's still using," she said. "Forget it, you two together? That's gasoline and a match. And your mom won't stop it."

I opened my mouth to argue, but she cut me off.

"I'm not raising our kids in a house with two addicts," she said. "I won't do it."

She turned away, back to the boxes, wiping her eyes as she packed. Her silence was louder than anything she could've yelled.

And right then, I knew I was about to lose a lot more than a house.

# 19

## DESTRUCTION

We moved out separately.

Chrissi took the kids and went to her parents' place. I moved into Mom and Dad's house. We split up the boxes like we were splitting up a life—half for her, half for me. She packed photos into two piles. "These are yours," she said, setting a stack on the counter. "For your new place." The rest went in a different box. For her place. I stood there staring at them, not knowing what to say. How do you divide a life like that? A home like that?

We'd moved into that big house as a family. Built it from the ground up. Now we were carrying boxes out of it like strangers. Broken. Maybe beyond repair.

We'd pulled the kids out of their private school—couldn't afford it anymore. Enrolled 'em in the same public school I'd gone to, back when life was simpler and nothing burned. I saw them as much as I could. Took them to school some mornings. Picked them up when Chrissi needed a break. Did what I could.

But I was living off $1,100 a month in disability. That's it. Barely enough for gas and groceries. Couldn't cover the rent or the insurance or school stuff. Best I could do was keep their cell phones turned on.

Chrissi never asked for more. She never yelled or blamed. Maybe she didn't have the energy left to.

I remember sitting on the edge of the mattress at my parents', holding a picture frame in my lap. One of those beach photos—us smiling like nothing could ever touch us. And I just kept thinking, *How did we get here?*

We hadn't just lost the house. Or the shop.

We'd lost the "we."

I'D HAD this one psychiatrist early on—he was also a lawyer, sharp guy. Knew the system, knew people, knew how to talk to somebody like me without making me feel like I was broken beyond repair. He was the only one I felt listened. But then he quit practicing. After that, I bounced around from one doctor to the next. None of them helped. And eventually, I stopped pretending they could.

But the insurance said I had to go. So, I did. Not because I believed help was coming—but because the mileage paid out. That's the truth. Back then, I wasn't going to doctors to get better. I was going so I could keep the pills coming—and so I could cash that mileage check from workers' comp. That check felt like a paycheck. Thirty bucks here, fifty there. Add it up over a month, it covered gas, snacks, and whatever I needed to make it through another day without falling apart.

I remember walking into the office of this new guy they set me up with. Same waiting room smell—bleach, fear, and bad coffee. I checked in, sat down, and already knew what I was gonna do: tell him what he wanted to hear, get my scripts, get my miles. That was the plan.

He called me back. He was a middle-aged guy with a slumped posture who wore his white coat like it was too heavy for him. He sat behind his desk with his pen in hand and asked me how I'd been doing.

I laid it out for him. Half-true. Just enough pain and stress to justify what I wanted. I talked about the accident. The pain. The nightmares. The anxiety. I left out the part about already being on pills. Just gave him the edited version.

He looked at me over his glasses, eyes soft. "Mr. Hardison," he said, voice low and full of pity. "I don't know what I would do if I were you. But we're going to give you some medication to help."

Then he started writing. Script after script.

Pain pills. Antidepressants. Sleep meds.

Then came the Xanax.

"These come in bars," he said. "But break them in half. Take half in the morning and half at night."

Sounded reasonable.

Except the script was for 60 pills. Thirty days. Do the math—he just told me to take one a day but gave me enough for two. And he knew that. I saw it. But I didn't say a word. Just folded the paper and slid it into my wallet like a winning lottery ticket.

I left that office floating.

For a while, I told myself this was still a treatment. Still medical. Still legit. But now? Now I look back, and I get mad. Mad at myself. Mad at that doctor. Mad at the whole broken system.

Those pills made me sleep almost all day, every day. I'd pass out in my recliner in the middle of the afternoon, drool on my shirt, the sound of cartoons in the background while my kids played without me. What kind of dad can you be if you're too drugged out to even stand up?

I thought I was managing it. Thought I was showing up.

Truth was, I wasn't showing up for anybody—not even myself.

I kept going every month to get new scripts. One day, the doctor left the room in a rush—something about needing to grab a chart or check on a patient down the hall. I was sitting there on that crinkly paper, foot tapping, fingers twitching, thinking about how long it'd been since my last dose.

And that's when I saw it.

The prescription pad. Just sitting there on the counter like an invitation.

I stared at it for a minute, heart thudding in my chest. Everything within me knew it was wrong. I knew better. But I also knew what it could do.

I reached over, slid it off the counter, and tucked it into my jacket pocket. Smooth. Quiet. No hesitation.

When the doctor came back, I acted like nothing had happened. Nodded, shook his hand, walked to the front desk, signed my name, and checked out like I always did.

Then I went home and got to work.

It wasn't like I wrote anything crazy. I knew the language, knew the dosages. I'd seen enough scripts in my life by that point to write one in my sleep. Made it look legit. Signed the doctor's name just like he did.

I didn't even try to fill them myself. That would've been stupid. Instead, I handed them to Dad.

"Take this in," I said. "Go to different pharmacies, OK? Rotate them. Never the same one more than once a month. You hear me?"

He nodded, slipped the folded paper into his wallet, and walked out the door.

I didn't explain why I gave him that warning. Maybe I should've. Or maybe he just didn't care. Either way, it worked for months. It allowed me to get the drugs I wanted without buying off the street. Still illegal. But safer. At least that's what I told myself.

But then, one day, Dad went back to Fred's—the same pharmacy he'd already been to that month. The same one we'd used not even two weeks before.

The lady behind the counter looked at the prescription and the name and began to ask questions.

"Excuse me," she told Dad, as she slipped into the back office.

He waited and tried to act normal. But he could feel it.

She called the doctor. "Yes, for Pat Hardison?"

"No," he said. "I haven't written him that prescription in months."

And just like that, it was over.

I hadn't just crossed a line—I'd stomped all over it. Felony forgery. Caught red-handed.

Thought I was smart enough to stay ahead and play the system. A system that is unforgiving. It doesn't care if you're a burn survivor or a former firefighter. Doesn't care how much pain you're in. Doesn't care about the excuses you've told yourself in the dark.

I was in trouble. Real trouble. And this time, there was no prescription that could make it go away.

## 20

# INTERVENTION

When the house of cards falls down around you, you become more willing to listen when people beg you to get help. Lori had been begging for years now, especially the last two years since Chrissi and I had separated, but she finally got me to agree to go to rehab.

"Chrissi," she said, the phone trembling in her hands, "he's finally agreed to go."

Chrissi didn't answer right away. On the other end of the line, Lori could hear her breathing. Kids laughing in the background. A dish clinked into the sink.

"Really? To rehab?" Chrissi finally asked.

"Yes," Lori said. "He'll have to see the psychiatrist first. But he's agreed. He's gonna do it."

Another long pause. Then Chrissi asked, quieter this time, "Is he serious this time?"

"As serious as I've seen him," Lori said. "He needs someone to take him to the appointment. And then straight to the facility. Would you take him?"

The line went silent again. Then Chrissi let out a sigh. "Alright. I'll take him."

. . .

When she came to pick me up, I said, "Know what today is? It's our tenth anniversary."

Chrissi glanced over at me, then back at the road. "I'm aware."

It had been seven years since my accident, and ten years since we said I do, and I wanted to mark the occasion. "Come on, let's go out to eat breakfast first before we go to the doctor. We don't know how long all this will take." And she agreed. I was putting off the inevitable and hopelessly trying to have one more day like Chrissi and I weren't living separate lives.

We drove to the psychiatrist's office in near silence. I stared out the window, watching the same streets I'd driven a hundred times before. But today felt different. Heavier. Chrissi didn't say much either, just gripped the steering wheel tight and kept her eyes on the road.

At the office, they called me back, and for once I told the truth. All of it. Told them about the pills, the forgery, the crash-and-burn spiral I'd been living in. It took a long time. Every word felt like I was pulling teeth out of my own mouth. Chrissi sat there the whole time, arms crossed, eyebrows raised, cautiously watching to see if I would lie.

We were there till almost 11:00 that morning before the psychiatrist finally closed his folder and leaned back.

"I'll make the recommendation," he said. "But you need to go straight there. No stops. No delays. From this office to the facility."

I nodded, then looked over at Chrissi. "It's our anniversary today."

He blinked. "Excuse me?"

"Ten years," I said. "Can we at least get lunch before I go in? One last meal together. I promise I'm going."

He hesitated. Looked at Chrissi. Then back at me. "Straight there after?"

"Yes, sir," I said. "No detours."

He finally nodded. "Okay. But don't make me regret it."

We left the office and drove to a restaurant nearby. Chrissi didn't say much, and I didn't blame her. I ordered soup and salad, something light. Something easy. But before we got there, I'd taken a handful of pills. I didn't even think twice. I knew they'd take everything from me at check-in, and I wasn't ready to give it up yet. I went out on my terms.

I barely remember the meal. Don't remember eating. Don't remember the check. All I remember is blacking out right there at the table, head slumped over next to my untouched bowl of soup. Chrissi reached across the table and touched my arm, trying to rouse me. The waitress hovered behind her, unsure of what to do. Chrissi didn't explain. Just slipped a few bills onto the table and somehow got me out the door.

By the time we pulled into the facility, I was high. Eyes glossy, body heavy, brain fogged over. But the staff didn't blink. If you weren't carrying the pills in with you, they didn't ask many questions. They just took your name and told you where to go. Detox was expected. Pain was assumed. Nobody cared how wrecked you were when you arrived as long as you made it through the door.

But what I didn't know was that this place wasn't rehab. Not technically. It was a psychiatric hospital. The kind of place for folks who couldn't tell what year it was. Patients who talked to people who weren't there. People brought in after suicide attempts or psychotic breaks. Most of them weren't there by choice.

There were a few detox cases. But not many.

And me? I was already planning my exit.

I'd come in on my own, which meant I could leave on my own. So, I did what any addict would do when the fog started lifting just enough to panic: I called home.

"Dad," I said into the phone. "Come get me."

He didn't ask questions. Said he'd be there soon. But apparently, he called Lori first.

"Chrissi probably hasn't even made it home yet. Why don't you call her and see if she will turn around and go get him?" Dad asked, not wanting to be the bad guy, but not wanting to drive all the way up there either.

"There's no way Chrissi will come back to pick him up," she told my parents. "Not after this. She's done."

Still, they tried to figure something out.

"Let me call his therapist," Lori said. "See if there's anything he can do before y'all go get him."

She got him on the phone. A soft-voiced man who had probably heard too many broken stories to be rattled by mine.

"Can't you make him stay?" Lori pressed. "He's high as a kite right now. He's not in his right mind. He's a danger to himself."

"I understand your concern," the therapist said, voice calm. Too calm. "But he came in voluntarily. If he wants to leave, he can."

Lori wasn't having it.

"Come on. You're telling me you can't do anything? Can't you take his shoes? His clothes? Lock a door, delay paperwork, something? Just long enough for him to detox and maybe think clearly for once?"

There was a pause.

"No, ma'am," the therapist finally said. "We can't do that."

Lori sighed, heavy and tired. "You're gonna let him walk out of there like this?"

"I don't have a choice."

And that was when she deployed the nuclear weapon in her arsenal. "Do you understand he's committed all these felonies now? He's stolen a prescription pad. He's written his own prescription for drugs. Insurance has caught up with him. All these things are going on and he has to get help!"

"You can call the sheriff and turn him in." Her lifeline.

. . .

But she didn't call the police, she called my dad back. "Dad, you have to do this. You have helped create this monster and now the only way to keep him safe is to turn him in to the Sheriff. If not, he will end up driving when he's out and either hurt himself or somebody else."

Dad got in his car and headed to the facility. I was thrilled, having no idea of all the calls that had been taking place behind the scenes. I got in his car, and we headed home, or so I thought.

But Dad had done as Lori told him. Called Brad Lance, Chief Deputy of Tate County Sheriff Department, and former classmate of mine. We had gone to school together, and now he would be in charge of locking me up.

As we got close to Senatobia, past the Tate County line, Dad pulled the car over to the side of the road. I saw the cruiser pull up behind us, no lights or sirens. I raised my eyebrows at my dad. "What's this all about?"

As I glanced in the rearview mirror, I saw her walking up on my side of the car, so I rolled down my window. "Hey, Lisa, what's up?" Sergeant Lisa Sanders. Another classmate. I had known her since we were kids. She had been in the grade below me at school. We had worked scenes together when I was still in the fire department. Now, here she was, at one of my lowest points, come to arrest me, I was sure.

"Hey, Pat. Hate to be meeting like this but you know there is a warrant out for your arrest. I'm going to need you to come with me."

I looked back at my dad. My stomach dropped. He wouldn't meet my eyes.

I stepped out of the car as my friend and former classmate handcuffed me on the side of the road and helped me into her patrol car.

"Here Pat, sit in the front." Lisa said, giving me at least that dignity. "I hate seeing you like this, man. We'll get you some help."

## 21

## DETOX

They gave me a private cell. Not because I asked but because I knew most of the guys running the jail, either through school or I had worked fires with them. But thinking you could be comfortable in jail is a joke. A private cell is still concrete and bars. It's still cold. Loud. Full of things you can't fix.

The first night, I started shaking. Skin crawling, muscles twitching like they were trying to leave my body. I was burning up and freezing at the same time. I threw up everything in my stomach, then dry-heaved until my throat was raw. My body begged for pills. Begged for anything.

THEN CAME THE SEIZURES.

The first one slammed into me in the middle of the night. I remember lying on that paper-thin mattress, sweating through my shirt, and then everything went black. I woke up to a guard pounding on the bars, yelling my name, his voice crackling through the fog in my brain.

"You alright, Pat? You with me?"

I couldn't speak. My mouth was dry as sand. I nodded once and curled back into myself. My muscles locked up again not long after that. I convulsed. Gritted my teeth so hard that I swore they cracked. They called the nurse, but there wasn't much she could do except stand there with her clipboard, and watch me ride it out.

Your body turns on you during detox. It screams, thrashes, twists, begs—anything to make you give it what it thinks it needs. There's no relief. No sleep. No breath that doesn't come with fire. Your skin hurts. Your bones ache. Your thoughts start to break apart.

You hallucinate. See shadows on the walls that aren't there. Hear voices. One night I thought I was in a war, and the guards were enemy soldiers. As I came out of the fog, I remembered that before I had agreed to go to the rehab facility, I had tried to convince Lori that I could detox at her place.

"Look, I'm not going to rehab, but you are right, I need to get off all this stuff. Why don't I come and stay in y'all's camper?"

"Uh…" Lori had hesitated, but I heard Clark's voice loud and firm in the background. "Absolutely not! He goes to rehab. That's the only option."

What if I had been there at their camper and all this had happened? With Clark's guns in their house? With their kids inside? Jail was awful. But it was safer—for everybody.

MY FAMILY CAME on the weekends. Brought food. Checked in. They asked the nurses at the local hospital if there was anything they could do. Something to ease the symptoms. But this was before Narcan was standard. There was nothing. The only way through was *through*.

I don't remember every detail. Just flashes. Sweat soaking through my shirt. My mom crying when she saw me. My dad trying to act like everything was fine, talking about the weather and football. Lori calling me and asking how I was doing.

She told me something one day that stuck with me. "The Bible talks about the potter and the clay," she said, "but it also talks about silver. You know how they purify silver, Pat? They heat it up until it melts. Until the impurities rise to the top. And then they scrape it clean."

I stared at the receiver on the wall.

"That's what this is," she said. "You're silver. And fire is the only way to refine silver. You're being refined."

AFTER THE WORST of the withdrawal passed, something in me snapped—I was angry at everybody.

Mad at the doctors who told me I needed the drugs. Mad at my dad for always keeping the supply coming. Mad at myself for swallowing it all down without asking a single question.

Now that the pills were gone, I felt fine. Not perfect. But at least I could function again. I could breathe better. I could think much more clearly.

And all I could think was—if I'd done this years ago, maybe we'd still have the house. Maybe I wouldn't have lost Chrissi. Maybe my kids would still see me as more than the guy who slept in the recliner all afternoon.

I've had major surgeries. Been burned alive. And I'd do all of that again before I'd choose to detox like that one more time.

That's how bad it was.

People say, "Just quit." They don't get it. This ain't about willpower. It's about your brain convincing your body that poison is the only way to survive.

I wasn't trying to get high. I just didn't want to feel like I was dying.

AFTER A FEW WEEKS, I finally saw a judge. Small courtroom. Gray walls. It felt more like a principal's office than a courtroom.

He looked over my file and then looked over at me. I swear, for a second, I saw something in his eyes that wasn't judgment—it was understanding.

He didn't throw the book at me. Could have. I'd committed a felony. Forgery. Drug fraud.

But he didn't.

He looked at me and said, "Mr. Hardison, you need help. Not prison."

He gave me probation. Ordered me into rehab. A real one this time. One that knew what addiction looked like on someone who wasn't the typical junkie.

With over 30 days in the county jail, and then another 30 days in a rehab facility that knew what they were doing, I finally got clean.

It wasn't because I was strong.

It was because a few people—Lori, the judge, and even the jailers who gave me that cell—were strong when I wasn't.

I USED to wish I'd done it differently. Detoxed in that rehab first. Done it the right way.

But I wouldn't have stayed. I would've left the second it got hard.

I had to be locked up. Had to hit the bottom so hard the only way out was up.

Now, when parents call me begging for advice, telling me their twenty-something year-old kid is in jail, I tell them the same thing every time.

"Leave him there. Let him sit. Let him sweat it out. Best thing for him."

Because sometimes...hell is what wakes you up.

And waking up is the only way you live.

# PART V
# THE MIRROR BREAKS

## 22

## SHATTERED PIECES

Rehab helped me clean the fog from the mirror, but I still couldn't face the image staring back at me. In some ways, the image I saw now was even harder to face. From firefighter to felon. From husband to ex. From businessman known around town, to the person on disability they talked about behind their menus when I walked into a restaurant. The years after rehab are mostly a blur. I was still struggling—trying to figure out who I was now. As a dad. As a man. As somebody who used to matter. I was just doing it clean and sober.

My eyesight had continued to deteriorate from my initial injuries to where I could no longer drive myself around as I once had. The loss of my eyelids in the fire meant that my eyes were getting worse every day. I could no longer get a haircut, pick up dinner, or show up for my kids without asking for help. I couldn't see, had no job, no real way forward. Just a face that scared people, an $1100 a month disability check, and parents who still had to take care of me.

That strips something from you. Manhood, maybe. Or at least the part of it that's tied to strength, independence, respect. This wasn't what being a man is supposed to look like—living in a small room at your parents' house.

When you lose your face, you lose more than how you look. You lose the way people treat you. The way they smile at you in the checkout line. The way a stranger holds a door open without thinking twice. The way a kid looks at you without fear.

Fear—that was the first reaction people had to me most days. And that messes with your head. It makes you wonder if maybe you really are the monster they see.

When Chrissi filed for divorce, thankfully she didn't fight to keep me from the kids. She could have—she had the reasons and evidence to do so. But she didn't. She knew how much I love my kids, and that they were really all I had left.

Though I hadn't lost my kids, for a while the pain and the pills had kept me from being the dad I wanted to be. The one that was different from my own. The dad that they could depend on to show up when they called. The dad that wouldn't embarrass them in front of their friends. Or the one that could help them start businesses and keep them running.

But I hadn't been that dad. I had followed in the very footsteps I hated.

"No, you can't go with Daddy right now, he isn't feeling well." I could still hear Chrissi say to our kids, an excuse to keep them from following me as I was headed out the door to get lost in the woods, and in my own thoughts of how much I hated what I had become. And though I finally had the pills out of my system, it didn't erase those years when they weren't. I couldn't change what I became, all I could do was try to not become that same guy again and give my kids an opportunity to get a better dad.

"Pat, I need you to get to the house. Dad's heart rate is really low." The phone call stopped me in my tracks. I hadn't been at home but had been planning to head back to celebrate my mom's birthday, which was that day.

"Uh, yeah" I cleared my throat. I could barely speak. "I'll get a ride and be right there." And though I got there as quickly as I could, by the time I walked in the door, he was already gone.

I hated not being there when he died, but we had known it wouldn't be long. He had been out of it for days, on so much morphine because of the progression of the disease, that he didn't even know who was in the room.

Dad had been diagnosed with cirrhosis of the liver the year after I left rehab and had been fighting the disease for the last two years. He was also dealing with heart issues. All of his years of drinking and then the pills had finally caught up to him.

One day at the house, he fell and broke his hip because the alcohol made him lose his balance. The doctors did a hip replacement and sent him home with pain meds. After taking the pills, he got out of bed and fell again, this time dislocating his hip. The doctors couldn't do anything for him. His heart couldn't handle another surgery. They sent him home in a hospital bed to live out the rest of his life. The boys and I would try to get him up out of the bed, because he would beg. But he could never put weight on that leg, so he would flop back into the reclining position of the hospital bed in their house, defeated and discouraged. That is where he was until that phone call, the day he died, in 2011.

Mom had been praying for his healing, but with a different result in mind than when she prayed for me. She wanted Dad to go home and be with the Lord because she saw how much pain he was in. Mom believed that complete healing in the arms of Jesus was the only thing that was going to cure it. It broke her heart that she would not get to go to Shannon's wedding in Florida, because she couldn't leave him. He had been her partner for over four decades, and she would not leave him at the end, not even for her baby boy's wedding. But when Dad passed, just weeks before the wedding, it allowed her the peace of mind that he was finally with the Lord, and she could be with her child as he started his next chapter.

The sad thing was, Dad had begun to turn his life around during those last few years. Whether from seeing my own journey, or his

Savior finally getting his attention, I will never know, but he began going to church again with Mom and started taking things seriously. That's why it hurt so bad seeing him drink and do pills all those years, because when I was younger, I saw a sign of a transformation starting to peak through, but then it was as if it wore off, or was eclipsed by the pain of the PTSD, I'm not sure which. It made me mad he allowed himself to do those things. Once I was in recovery from the pills, I could look back on both of our lives and understand better than most why he had succumbed to those demons.

He wasn't perfect, but he was still my dad. *Why was I losing him now?* I had no house, no wife, family falling apart, now this? It felt as if something inside me was shattering. As the older son, you are supposed to be the one who steps up when something like this happens. You're expected to become the head of the family, take care of your mom and siblings, and shoulder the weight he had been carrying. But maybe that weight had been shouldered more by my mom all along. Just like Chrissi had carried the weight for so many years in our family until she finally set it down.

I felt more alone than ever. No amount of company changed it. Chrissi brought the kids to stay with me. Friends showed up consistently to take me to appointments. But something was missing, and I didn't know how to express it. I just went through the motions around people. I appreciated when they sat with me on the hard days and ate dinner with me like it was normal. They were trying to help me hold on to the man I used to be. But my smiles and laughs around others were fake. I wasn't ungrateful—I was just numb. I was trying to make people feel comfortable. Maybe Chrissi had been right with what she had said years prior. Maybe I really had died in the fire. The Pat before no longer existed.

A YEAR LATER, I was riding to a doctor's appointment with Clay Moore. Just the two of us in his truck, headed down the interstate. Clay always had some kind of music playing, usually gospel. This morning, he had it turned down more than usual.

"I saw something on TV last night," he said, keeping his eyes on the road. "Some doctor—Rodriguez, I think was his name. They were talking about a face transplant he and his team had just done on this guy in Baltimore. He's done some pretty incredible stuff," Clay went on. "Changed this guy's life. Said they take the donor's whole face—skin, muscle, everything—lift it off like it's a mask, and then fit it over the other guy's face and bone structure. Hook up all the blood vessels so it works like it's his own." He shook his head as if he still couldn't believe it. "And I couldn't stop thinking about you."

I didn't say anything right away. Just stared out the window, watching the fields blur by.

Clay glanced over at me. "Would you ever consider something like that? I mean, it sounds like you'd look like the guy you got the face from. You might not even like how you look."

I shrugged. "Well, hell, I know I wouldn't look like I do now!"

Clay wasn't the only one who had done research. I had found out in my darker days that with facial injuries like mine, the suicide rate is sky-high. Over eighty percent of patients who have both a physical deformity and functional deficits, like I did, have severe depression.[1] That's not a typo. That's the truth. We can't look in the mirror. Can't face the stares, the pain, the loss. The transplant wouldn't be just about looks—it's about restoring your sense of personhood. Your ability to look in the mirror and not see some shattered, broken thing staring back at you. I was willing to risk it all for that chance.

WE SAT in the eye doctor's office, with him examining my chronically dry eyes, shining lights in each one and asking the same questions he had asked many times before, "Pat, I hate to tell you, but your eyesight is still going downhill. If we can't figure out a way to protect your eyes without you having any eyelids, and get some moisture restored, you are looking at the very real possibility of going blind in a few years. That is the function of blinking—to clear debris and

---

1. https://www.sciencedirect.com/science/article/abs/pii/S0278239118301277

moisten your eyeballs. Without the ability to blink, you will eventually go blind."

Clay looked over at me, as though judging my reaction and seeking permission to dive off the deep end. "I was telling Pat on the way up here about this thing I saw on TV last night, a guy had a full face transplant. Have you ever heard of that?"

The doctor leaned back, folded his arms. "I saw an article recently. It's so new," he said. "I don't think there have been but a handful ever done and the success rates weren't great, so I really couldn't say if it would work. I wouldn't get your hopes up."

"But what about blinking?" I asked. "With a face transplant, wouldn't I then be able to blink again? To keep my sight?"

He hesitated. "To my knowledge, no one's ever had that restored, but as I said, I don't know much about the procedure."

He didn't mean to shut it down, but I walked out of that office feeling like I'd just asked for the moon and been told I was crazy.

# PART VI
# THE MAN I BECAME

# 23

# A MAN

A few days later, my phone rang, some strange number I didn't recognize, but I answered anyway. "Hello, my name is Dr. Eduardo Rodriguez. I am calling to speak to Mr. Pat Hardison?"

"This is he." I tried to keep my voice calm. I knew that name. Rodriguez. It had been stuck in my head every night since Clay first told me about him. Clay had said he might email the doctor, just to see, but I figured it was one of those things you talk about and never hear back. I sure hadn't done anything to follow up. Still, I'd been praying for a miracle. And now here he was.

"Pat, it's good to get you on the phone. Let me get straight to the point. I got an email from a friend of yours, a Mr. Clay Moore, telling me about your situation. That you were a firefighter. That you were burned in a house fire and lost most of the skin on your face and shoulders?"

"Yes, sir." My heart felt like it was going to pound out of my chest.

"As he may have told you, I'm a plastic surgeon who specializes in facial reconstruction. We recently had success with a full facial transplant, and I'd love to talk to you about the possibility of you having the same surgery. Now, before I get your hopes up—there will be many hoops to jump through. First, I'll need your medical records from the past two years..."

He kept going, carefully explaining all the steps. Telling me there were no guarantees. Said that even if we did everything right, I still might not be a match. But my brain was already a mile ahead. I was picturing kids smiling at me again. Watching my boys play ball without people staring. The sound of his voice started to fade as the sound of hope got louder.

"...so get your medical records released to me for the past two years plus from your initial accident, and I will review them. Does that sound good?"

"Yes, sir. Absolutely."

"Great, we'll be in touch."

"Sounds good."

I hung up and just sat there for a minute, trying to breathe. This surgery—this miracle—might actually be a possibility. I just had to get some records together. I could do that.

THE LADY behind the counter tapped her keyboard a few times, then gave a low whistle.

"This is a big file," she said.

I just nodded. "I was here for a while."

She kept scrolling. "You were in the burn unit for... how long?"

"Sixty-three days."

She looked up at me again, this time slower. "That'll explain it."

She printed off the release forms and slid them across the counter. "You'll need to fill these out, sign here, and initial here. We'll send the records once we process them."

"Good," I said. "Send 'em wherever they need to go."

She hesitated. "There's going to be a charge."

"Okay. How much?"

"We charge $0.50 per page. It looks like you've got over a thousand pages here, maybe closer to two."

I didn't flinch. "Can I call you back with a credit card number?"

Burn unit records add up fast. Three nurses a day, each writing notes every shift. Vitals logged around the clock. Medications tracked, reactions recorded, specialists brought in. Every surgery, every scan, every IV. Every time somebody changed a bandage or cleaned a wound. All of it documented. Stacked up like layers on a tree stump—each one marking what it took to keep me alive.

That was the cost of surviving.

Was it expensive? Yeah. Over $500 just to copy it all and send it off.

If there was a chance this doctor could help me see, help me blink, help me live—then I'd pay whatever it took.

Hell, I'd have sold the tires off my truck if I had to.

She took my signed paperwork and started stamping dates and filing things away. Then she paused. "I want to make sure you realize, Mr. Hardison, that this release is just for your records here at The Med," she said. "If that doctor needs files from any coordinating physicians—surgeons, specialists, physical therapy—you'll have to go to each of their offices separately. They'll have their own forms and fees."

I just stared at her for a second. "You're tellin' me this ain't even all of it?"

She gave a little shrug. "Hospital records only cover what happened inside these walls. Anything outpatient or from a private practice is on you."

I nodded. Of course it was.

I thanked her and headed out. The air outside hit me like a wall—hot, thick, and sticky. I climbed into the car and just sat there for a second, leaving the engine idling. There would now be another round of phone calls. Another week of chasing down signatures and fax numbers. Another set of hoops to jump through, just like Dr. Rodriguez had warned me.

But I'd come this far.

And I wasn't stopping now.

APPARENTLY ABOUT THE same time that Clay was emailing Dr. Rodriguez, my eye doctor had gone down to New Orleans for a medical conference. Professional development, networking. New Orleans is just a few hours south on Interstate 55. Easy trip. Plus, let's be honest, it's not a bad place to spend a few days.

One of the keynote speakers that year was none other than a plastic surgeon named Dr. Eduardo Rodriguez. My doctor told me later how this surgeon walked on stage—calm, collected, confident—and started talking about surgeries most people in that room had only read about in journals. Cutting-edge stuff. Face transplants. Surgical firsts. New frontiers in medicine.

Somewhere in the middle of that talk, something must've clicked for my doctor. After it ended and people started to drift out, he made his way to the front. Reached into his jacket, pulled out a business card, flipped it over, and wrote my name on the back in those small, blocky letters I'd recognize anywhere.

When he got his chance, he stepped up and said, "Dr. Rodriguez, I've got a patient I want you to talk to. I think you could help him."

Rodriguez nodded politely, took the card, and slipped it into his pocket with all the others people had handed him that day. He flew back to Baltimore the next morning. Business as usual. But when he walked into his office, my medical records were sitting there on his desk. He pulled out the stack of cards from the conference, started flipping through them—and there was my name on top. Same name as on those records.

He told me later it felt like divine confirmation. That I was meant to be his next patient.

"HEY, PAT," Dr. Rodriguez began. My records had been with him for a few weeks, and I had been eagerly waiting for his call. "I have reviewed your records and would like to begin the process of getting approval for the surgery."

"Awesome, I'm ready. How soon can we do it?" I was eager to get moving. I had been waiting for this for eleven years.

"Hang on, Pat. As I told you before, this is not the same as the surgeries you have had in the past where the doctors determine this is the best course of action and you agree and everything moves forward. We need to begin with tests to determine what can be done and what cannot. There are no guarantees that this will work, and I need you to be clear on that before we even get started."

That's how he talked. Straightforward. No fluff. No false hope.

I know he wasn't just being a medical professional, and I could tell that he actually cared. I appreciated that, but I'd already made up my mind. This was going to work. Period.

"I hear you, Doc, so just tell me how to get started."

"I love your enthusiasm, Pat. It may just be the difference in the outcome. I will have the appointment desk call you with a time to fly up here and have the first round of tests. There'll be standard blood tests," he said, "but we'll also need to do detailed scans of every structure in your face. Then you and I will sit down together and go over the whole process. I know you're eager to get started, but there's still a lot you don't know. We need to talk through it carefully so that we're both sure you're making the right call. For example—there's only about a fifty percent chance you survive the surgery, Pat. This has only been done a handful of times, and never to the extent we're talking about here. If you've got any doubts—any at all—after hearing that, I need you to tell me."

"I'm 100% a go, Doc." See, I never had a doubt, not once. I couldn't let my mind go there. I'd already lived through hell. The only option was that this worked. *It had to. It will.*

WEEKS LATER, I was sitting across from Dr. R in a conference room in Baltimore at the University of Maryland Medical Center, discussing the details of the surgery. "Pat, I am honored that you are willing to consider this possibility. Because this is an experimental surgery, the costs are being covered by the hospital, so you don't have to worry about that..."

"Out of curiosity, how much does a surgery like this cost?"

"Easily over a million dollars." He didn't blink at that number. As if these were numbers he spoke about every day.

"Whew. OK. Glad that won't be *my* bill."

"No, Pat, but understand that the cost to you might be even higher, including possibly paying with your life."

I shook my head. "Not going to happen."

"Ok, Pat, I hear you. Let's discuss the tests that we will need to do to make sure that your body is compatible with the procedure, and that you can handle everything that will be involved."

What was involved began with a year and a half of tests. Psychological evaluations, physical assessments, interviews. They had to evaluate me—my mind, my will to live, whether I could handle the weight of what I was asking for. I was flying back and forth to Baltimore regularly as they would review the results of one set of tests and order more. They were trying to figure out if I had what it took to survive—not just the surgery, but the life afterward.

THE COLD STERILE air of the conference room was of little comfort as Dr. R shifted to his next item on the agenda of our discussion during that first trip to meet him. "Pat, we're not releasing anything to the press. Not yet."

I nodded. "Good. I don't want it out there either."

Truth was, I didn't need the world watching me while I laid there looking like roadkill, hoping for a miracle. And I *sure* didn't want my kids hearing about some new development in my case on the news before I could explain it to them myself.

By then, my youngest was ten. Old enough to understand. Old enough to hear a headline or catch something on TV and start asking questions I couldn't answer yet.

What if it didn't work?

What if I died?

Or worse, I lived, but it was worse than before?

That's not how I wanted them to find out. Not from a stranger with a microphone.

I'd already missed too much with them. Missed school pickups and games and birthdays, just trying to survive. I wasn't about to let the media steal this too.

We kept it quiet. Just between family and the folks who needed to know.

Not that they were that excited about this surgery, mind you. In fact, they thought I'd lost my mind. Why would I take this risk? Was I so lost that I didn't actually care whether I lived through the surgery?

"Dad, why do you even want to do this? You're perfect to us." Cullen didn't like it one bit.

I just shook my head. "I'm not, though. I want to look normal when I stand next you at your wedding, when I hold your kids."

But I could still see it in his eyes—the fear. Not of what I looked like now. But of losing me completely.

All of them were scared. And I don't blame them. To them, I was just *Dad*. They didn't see the burns. They didn't flinch when they hugged me. Never once hesitated to touch my face. For the younger two—I'd looked like this their whole lives. This was the only version of me they'd ever known.

They loved me exactly as I was.

They didn't need me to be fixed. They just needed me *here*.

To them it felt like a gamble they wouldn't have taken. A risk they didn't ask for.

But to me? It was the only way forward.

I wasn't trying to die. I was trying to live. *Without this working, how else would I be able to truly do that?*

"After we run all the tests here, we still need to make sure that you have the right support system back home." Dr. R was continuing down his list of topics that first day in Baltimore. Topics we needed to discuss before I could even get approved. His pen tapping on the legal pad laying in front of him on the conference table.

"I would like to come down to Mississippi and meet everyone, see for myself that you have a group around you that will be there when it gets hard. Because Pat, I know you say you are ready, but it will get hard. And what will make the difference is who you have around you when it does. I cannot emphasize enough the experimental nature of this surgery. We cannot guarantee its outcomes. All we can do is control everything that is within our power, such as making sure you have the right support."

"Sure, Doc, you are welcome anytime."

It took close to two years for all the tests that needed to be completed in Baltimore before Dr. Rodriguez flew down to Mississippi to see for himself. He wanted to meet everybody. My family. My friends. The guys at the firehouse.

I called everyone on a Thursday night and told them, "Hey, I'm having a face transplant and the doctor is flying down and wants to meet everyone. Be at the house Sunday, we are going to have a big party."

"What are you even talking about?" most responded, shock filling their voice. I hadn't been telling people what was going on, as we had agreed. I had been holding this card close to my chest for a year, and not just because I had agreed to, but because it felt like if I told people, then it might not happen. But now, I was so far in that nothing could stop this procedure.

Friends, family, and my brothers from the force all knew now, and they showed up to meet the doctor.

We welcomed Dr. R the only way we knew how. Crawfish boil and a trip to the firehouse. Steaks on the grill. Stories around the table. Pictures from before—of me as a kid, as a young recruit to the force, holding my babies.

While Dr. R was down here in Mississippi, we drove to the location where the fire had taken place. The original house had of course been torn down and a new one built in its place. A perfect metaphor for the tearing down of my old, scared face and replacing it with a new donor one.

The night before he left to head back to Baltimore, Dr. R. looked me in the eye and said, "Pat, I've been offered the chair of plastic surgery at NYU Langone." He waited for my reaction, but I was waiting to see what this meant for me. "I'm dedicated to you. I gave you my word. If you want to stay in Baltimore, I'll stay. I'll see this surgery through with you before I make the move."

He paused, like he was weighing every word. "But if you're willing, we could go to New York. The chances of finding a donor match are better there. It's your call."

I didn't have to think long. We were two years into this thing already. I said, "Doc, you tell me where I need to be, and I'll be there." What did it matter to me where the surgery took place?

He took the job in New York, and I followed him.

I thought the hardest part was behind me. I'd done the tests, the evaluations, everything they asked. I figured when Dr. R moved to New York, we'd pick up right where we left off.

Wrong.

None of it transferred. Not the paperwork. Not the approvals. Nothing. State to state, hospital to hospital—it was like starting from scratch. Different laws. Different systems. Different hoops.

We had to climb the same mountain all over again.

The only difference was—I wasn't stumbling blindly this time. I knew the terrain. I knew what to expect. This was going to be an experimental surgery, funded by the hospital, and they had to be sure. Every test had to be double-checked. Every report, re-evaluated.

And that was okay.

Frustrating as hell. Slow as molasses. But I had something now I hadn't had in years. A plan. A shot. A reason to believe I could be the man I used to be.

DR. R TURNED towards me in the padded conference chair, his hands coming to rest on the conference table. Looking back, I can see how he was trying to be clear with me in that first meeting in Baltimore—not to let me think this surgery was going to be my salvation. "Pat, please understand, you can do everything right, get all the tests done, have all the right evidence, and the hospital still decide not to continue with the surgery. That is their right to say yes or no, and we will have to accept that. They won't make that decision lightly, so please understand that their call will be final."

I nodded. I couldn't imagine that would actually happen, but what else could I do? I would jump through all their hoops, answer all their questions, and let that be that. I couldn't imagine God would deny me the surgery after showing me this hope.

I HAD BEEN a man on a mission for two years, doing everything asked of me, twice now by two different hospitals, when I finally got the call I had been dreaming of.

"Pat, the surgery is a go—as long as we can find a donor," Dr. Rodriguez told me. "LiveOnNY is the coordinating agency. Keep a bag packed. Be ready. When we get the call, there won't be much time.

## 24

# A SON

"Would you like some water?" the assistant asked as she stepped into the conference room. She set bottles on the table and began refilling the snack trays, moving with the quiet efficiency of someone who knew we'd been at it for over an hour—and weren't close to done.

It was that first meeting with Dr. R in Baltimore. We'd already covered what the process would look like from start to finish, and now he was easing into the part I'd been both waiting for and dreading—the details of the surgery itself.

"I'm good," I told her.

Dr. R shook his head, indicating he didn't need anything either, then turned toward the screen at the end of the room. A projection flickered to life; presentation slides queued up to walk me through exactly what would happen.

"Pat, this surgery will not be like transplanting a kidney or liver. Matching the blood type is the easy part. What we need is a match for everything else. Bone structure. Skin tone. The space between your eyes. The shape of your nose. Even how your lips sit on your face. Everything needs to line up," he said. I just kept nodding, just going through the hoops of the verbal warnings, refusing to accept any potential complications. He continued. "We screen the donor for everything—no cancer, no facial injuries, no heavy drug use. Even tattoos can disqualify a donor because they can carry risks of contamination. This has to be a clean match. Inside and out."

"That narrows down the field of donors quite a bit then, doesn't it?" I said.

"Yes, Pat, it does. First, a coordinating agency will help us find a donor. Next, the donor's family will have to agree to donate. It's not like we're asking a parent for their deceased child's kidney, or even a heart, which might be easier for them to agree to. We will be asking a parent for their son's entire face."

I sat there for a minute as that sank in. I thought about my mom. How many times she'd prayed for me, that I would be healed and restored. How many nights she'd sat with me, helpless, wishing she could fix it.

I was still her son. Burned, broken—but hers. And now I would have to wait for another mom to lose her son for my mom's prayers to be answered.

"It might take months, even years, to find a donor who fits all the criteria and whose family agrees." Dr. R never wanted me to get my hopes too high.

It took two years from that first meeting in Baltimore to even get on the transplant list. Once I officially got approved, I would wake up every morning thinking—*maybe today's the day.*

I prayed.

This wasn't about vanity. It was about being able to eat without pain. About opening my mouth without my skin tearing. About walking into a room with kids laughing at my antics instead of staring in fear.

It was about breathing easier. Blinking. Keeping what little vision I had left.

It was about dignity.

And every day they didn't find a match, I kept reminding myself—God didn't bring me this far just to leave me here.

But my optimism clashed with the sad reality.

For me to live with a new face, someone else had to die.

It wasn't like praying for a job or a check to come in the mail. This was different. I was out here begging God for a miracle that could only come after heartbreak. A son. A brother. Maybe even a dad—gone. A family wrecked. Somebody's worst day. That was a necessary part of God answering my prayer—and I hated it. I felt greedy. Like I was asking too much.

I had to pull myself back and calm the part of me that wanted it so bad I couldn't breathe.

"God," I'd whisper, "help me not be selfish. Help me wait the right way. I hate that this comes at the cost of someone else's pain. Let it be the right one. Please be with that family."

AND THEN?

NOTHING.

MONTHS PASSED.

THANKSGIVING CAME—NOTHING.

CHRISTMAS—STILL NOTHING.

I TRIED to keep hope alive, but after a while, it started to get quiet inside. Not the peaceful kind of quiet either—instead, it was a more disruptive kind. More like doubt sneaking in dressed as silence. Dr R's prediction about it taking months had come true, and it was looking like it might even take years.

When spring rolled around a call from Dr. Rodriguez finally

came in. I waited on the other end of the line listening to him speak. *Please tell me something good, Doc.* A feeling of nausea hit me as I waited for the news.

"Pat, we've got a match. We're 98% sure. You need to get up here."

I almost forgot what peace felt like after all those years, but there it was. Gentle. Reassuring. Soothing. That feeling of peace hugged me like a child refusing to let go of their parents.

"Pat are you there?" he asked.

"Yes, sir. See you in New York, Doc." *This is real. This is going to happen. And absolutely nothing is going to stop it!*

THEY ARRANGED a private plane out of a small airport in Batesville, just a few miles south of Senatobia. A few of my buddies came with me—men who'd been by my side since the beginning. We flew to Meridian, picked up my sister Lori, then headed to New York. It was probably ten or eleven at night when we landed. After sitting in that hotel, all of us unable to sleep and wired with anticipation for the next move, we heard the phone ring. They said they needed me to come in for some lab work. I figured that meant things were moving. But then, around two in the morning, they called again. This time they said they needed one more test. *Something wasn't right*, I thought. I looked over at Bill and said, "It ain't gonna happen." I could feel it in my gut. That quiet drop in your stomach when hope starts slipping through your fingers.

After all the tests were done, they eventually told me more about the donor. He was Latino. Dark hair. Tan skin. I'm as Irish as they come—pale as a sheet, burn in the shade. It wasn't about looking like my old self—I'd let go of that a long time ago—but I didn't want to come out looking like a completely different person. Not when I was already unrecognizable. Still, I was so desperate, I tried to talk myself into it. Maybe skin tone wouldn't matter. Maybe people would just be glad I had a nose again. But deep down, I knew—I wasn't just being given a new face. I'd be carrying a piece of somebody's son. And it needed to feel right. Like something I could live with—and live up to.

Even if I could talk myself into it, I still had my family with their opinions and plain speech that never held back punches. Lori wasn't having it. She spun around in that hospital room, gave me one of those looks only a sister can give, and said, "Pat, you are not Latino. You're Irish. You're white as snow. You're gonna look like a quilt." I laughed, but deep down I knew she was right.

In the end, it didn't matter. The donor's family said no. They were Catholic, strong in their faith, and they just couldn't bring themselves to say yes—not for something like this, not to a stranger. I respected that. Truly. But it still knocked the wind outta me.

The ride back to the hotel was dead quiet. I wanted to scream, throw something, anything to get the weight off my chest. But I didn't. I just sat there, holding the disappointment. That was our first false run. My first *almost*. And it stung.

I'd been so sure it was happening. I'd let myself believe it. Although it was disappointing, Lori reminded me, like she always did, that you can't force God's timing. If this one wasn't right, then it just meant the right one hadn't come yet.

We went back to Mississippi to reset, repack the bag, and wait. Again.

THE SECOND TIME THEY CALLED, it was early summer. June, maybe July. I remember the heat.

"Mr. Hardison," they said, "we've got another possible donor. We're gonna wait and see how it plays out."

I didn't even flinch. Just told them, "Look, I'm ready to get this over with. Just tell me when to be there."

But we never even made it to New York. That one didn't work out either.

When the phone rang again in August, I figured it was another false alarm. That's how this stuff went—my hopes would get up and then they would get crushed. I almost didn't answer, but I had to.

"Same hair color. Skin tone. Everything's looking identical."

I hung up, sat there for a second, before calling my sister. "I'm heading up alone. I'll be back tomorrow. It's probably nothing."

Bill was out on the road driving his rig when I called him. "Man, don't go without me," he said. "I can be there in an hour."

I told him there wasn't any need. I was treating it like the other times. Quick trip. In and out. He didn't like it, but he understood.

My sister wasn't having it.

"You are not going up there without me," she said. "You *will* have that plane stop and pick me up."

So, I did.

We landed in Meridian, and she met me on the tarmac, just the two of us. No big send-off. No cameras. Just us and that little jet, sitting there quietly and gleaming like it was waiting for something, too.

It felt different this time.

Still unsure. Still holding our breath. But there was something in the air—like maybe, *just maybe*, this one would stick.

She snapped a picture of the plane and posted it on Facebook. Nothing loud. Just a simple, "If you know, you know. Start praying that this is the answer."

When we landed in New York, Dr. Rodriguez was there, waiting at the gate. That was different.

He looked me square in the eye and said, "This is 100% a go."


DAVID RODEBAUGH WAS 26 years old, riding his bike home from work in Brooklyn when he swerved to avoid a pedestrian. He wasn't wearing a helmet. The crash left him with injuries he couldn't survive.

A New York transplant from Ohio, David was a BMX racer and bike enthusiast. The year before, he'd won a Red Bull-sponsored race. He had a tight-knit group of friends who called each other brothers. Reminded me of the brotherhood I had with the guys on the force. He was a son with a devoted mother, like mine. And—most importantly, not just for me, but for four other families who would receive the gift of life—he had checked "organ donor" on his driver's license.

When LiveOnNY reached out to David's mom, Nancy, she didn't hesitate. She wanted her son to live on. To help someone else.

What's wild is—she understood the weight of it in a way most people wouldn't. Years earlier, she'd gone through facial reconstruction herself, after a car wreck. She knew what it was like not to recognize your own reflection. So, when they told her about me—that I was a firefighter, that I'd been waiting for this chance—she said it gave her peace. Said me being a firefighter told her I had the strength to handle the surgery.

The doctors showed us a picture of David. I remember Lori looking at it, then looking at me. "Pat," she whispered, "he looks like he could be our younger brother." And he did. Same hair color. Same skin tone. Same bone structure. For a transplant like this to work, the donor's features must line up within just a few millimeters. Somehow, his did.

It was almost hard to believe. After all that waiting and all those false starts, we finally had a match. Thank God for the brave mom that had said yes to an amazing and heart-breaking gift. As Dr. R had said when I got off the plane, it was 100% a go. And I was ready. *Was this God's timing that Lori was talking about? It had to be because if it wasn't, I didn't know if I could handle another disappointment.*

## 25

# A PERSON

Dr. R explained each step of the process in detail. "There will only be a short window of time for the transplant to take place, or the face will be useless. When you get to hospital, we will have only a few hours to get you into surgery."

*Finally,* I thought, *something that sounded fast!* We had been sitting in that conference room that first day in Baltimore for what felt like hours, and this was the first time Dr. R said something that sounded quick after painstakingly explaining all the ways that this process could take a really long time.

IT WAS AROUND three in the afternoon when Dr. Rodriguez met us at the airport in New York the day we got the call that all that waiting might be over. No buildup. No big speech. Just a quick, steady order: go eat something and be back at the hospital by six. That was it. One minute I was in Mississippi, bag still packed from the last false alarm. The next, I was in New York, being told to get ready for a surgery that might kill me—or save my life.

With uncertainty in the air and a few hours to kill in the Big

Apple, I did what any Mississippi boy would do before getting a new face. I went and ate a steak.

We found this little diner close to the hospital, nothing fancy. I sat there with Lori, picking at my meal, trying to act like this was just another Thursday. Truth was, I couldn't taste a thing. My stomach was too tight to eat much, but I kept pushing food around my plate anyway, pretending everything was normal. It was a strange feeling. I watched life go on for others, without knowing if mine was about to end or begin. On the outside, there was still traffic flowing. Still people walking by. Still servers topping off coffee like it was any other afternoon. For them, it probably was. For me, it was the edge of everything. On the inside, I was dwelling harder on the reality that I was about to undergo one of the biggest surgeries ever attempted.

IT HAD BEEN three years before, in that conference room in Baltimore, when Dr. R described to me for the first time how long the surgery would take and the intricacies involved. "You aren't the first person to go through a face transplant. My team has done this before. The idea first appeared in an article in 2002."

*A year after my accident*, I thought.

"At the time, it sounded more like science fiction than medical science. Then in 2005, a woman in France became the first to actually have the surgery. After that, there were a few others in various countries. Currently, only eight face transplants had ever been done in the United States, including one here. But this will be the first to include a full face and scalp. The first to attempt to restore blinking. People still argue about whether even offering this surgery is the right thing to do. Whether the risks are too high…" Dr. R continued.

I couldn't help but stare in silence as he spoke. As a firefighter you learn to put your trust in your partners. There are sometimes where you have to just let go and have faith that your buddy you're going in with is going to make sure you get out of the building alive. I may not have worn the uniform anymore, but I was facing another big fire. This time, my partner was Dr. R. I had to trust him. It's not like he gave me a reason not to, but it's not easy putting your life in the hands of somebody you barely know. He read off his track record as if that was the thing to assure me he was capable. No, that wasn't it. It was my intuition. I knew he was a guy who could get the job done. My thoughts were interrupted.

"Is any of this scaring you?" Dr. R asked, perhaps seeing my thousand-yard stare.

I shook my head. "No, sir." I didn't tell him I didn't care about the *how* of the surgery that much. I wanted to know things he couldn't tell me, like what it would feel like when I woke up. If I would recognize myself—or if anyone else would. When would I go back to being just Pat?

Now, here I was in New York, getting prepped for the surgery. I had to take a shower with a special antibacterial soap. Dried off and sat there on the gurney, as if awaiting a tone to drop for a fire I hadn't been on in years.

Nurses came in, asking if I was ready. I told them the same thing I'd been saying: "I was ready when Dr. R first called me about this surgery three years ago."

I'm not good at waiting. Never have been. When I say I'm ready, I mean it. Let's get it done. And when I make up my mind, there is no changing it.

I pulled the physical therapist aside, told him, "Hey, when this is over and y'all say I can get up—don't baby me. I don't care if it's only been one day, two days—if I am allowed to get up, you get me outta that bed." I hadn't come this far to lie here and feel sorry for myself. I came to get better. To get back to my kids. To live.

This wasn't just a physical fight—it was mental, emotional, and spiritual. Every part of me had to show up ready. There wasn't room for doubt and fear. I'd made peace with whatever might happen on that table, but still, I wasn't going in to lose.

. . .

THEY WHEELED me back just after dark. No turning back now. I gave Lori a nod. No big goodbye. No tears. Just that quiet look between people who've already said what needs saying. Others got the call—that the surgery was really happening, and happening fast. Everyone scrambled to get to New York. They met Lori, and Shannon once he arrived, in the waiting room and settled in beside them...to wait, and to pray. It would be over 24 hours later before they would be wheeling me back out of that OR to recovery.

"I WANT you to understand the enormity of this operation, Pat." Dr. R had told me during our first conversation in Baltimore. "It will take over one hundred people—surgeons, nurses, therapists, anesthesiologists, technicians, even an ethics team. We have spent years getting everyone ready. Training, planning, rehearsing like it was a NASA launch. We have practiced on cadavers to make sure we get it right. The whole hospital will be ready to move the second they got word about a donor." Dr. R's team in Baltimore had done the surgery before. Not so in New York. This was the very first facial transplant to be done in the state, much less at this facility. But the team had been training for years, with all the same precautions and preparations Dr. R had told me about in Baltimore.

ON THE NIGHT of my surgery, two operating rooms were running at the same time. One team worked on David, carefully removing his face and scalp. But first, they stopped and took a minute of silence to honor David and his family's sacrifice.

The other team started preparing me—removing what was left of my face and scalp. The teams worked in a coordinated dance, my team not removing any part from my face until they knew that part had been successfully removed and was viable from David's. Yet, they had to keep everything intact, so that the doctors could lay David's face over my skull like putting on a mask. It took over 8 hours for this part of the surgery alone.

When the time came, they brought the new face in. But this wasn't gluing a new face over an old one. They had to hook up muscles. Blood vessels thinner than a piece of thread. All of it had to be lined up just right so I could move my face, feel it, live in it. Blink. Dr. Rodriguez and his team didn't just give me a new face—they gave me an entire scalp with hair. They transplanted eyelids that could blink. Real ears. Pieces of bone from the donor—parts of the chin, the cheeks, the whole nose. They didn't just stitch skin. They rebuilt my entire head.

THE DONOR's face was without blood for three hours while being attached to me. Dr. R later said in an interview that his heart was racing as he tried to make sure each vessel was connected, knowing he couldn't relax until my face turned pink. That color was the sign that blood from my veins had started flowing into what would become my new face. If that color didn't appear, all of this would be in vain—the sacrifice of David's family, my family's prayers, everything. And it wouldn't be just David's family burying a son, but mine as well.

Near the end, they started seeing signs it was working. My new lips and ears—they turned pink. Life was moving through the new tissue. It wasn't just stuck on—it was becoming *me*.

I hadn't had real ears since the fire. Mine had been burned clean off. What I'd worn for years were those prosthetics I would tease the kids with—little snap-on ears that I stuck to magnets implanted in my head. They didn't feel like part of me. They didn't move. They didn't catch sounds right. They were just for show.

But these? These were alive. Warm. Pink with new blood. Flesh, bone, and feeling. They were a part of me now.

THE EYELIDS WERE A BIG DEAL. Before the surgery, mine were reconstructed pieces of skin, not working lids that could blink and clean and hydrate my eyes. Not having them, I was slowly going blind. They told me if something didn't change, I'd lose my sight altogether. And without blinking, I couldn't drive. Couldn't protect my eyes from dust or light or anything. I was losing my independence one little blink at a time.

But that day, they gave me back my blink.

It may seem like a small thing on the surface, compared to the nose or ears that you see when you look at a person, but those little working pieces of skin and muscle were the biggest breakthrough in the surgery. When you haven't been able to blink in years? When your eyes burn and ache all day and you can't even close them all the way at night? That blink is everything. And that particular procedure had never been done on a seeing patient before.

This surgery pushed the line. It changed what people thought was possible. This surgery didn't just change my life. It made it possible for doctors to change the lives of other patients after me.

## 26

# A FIGHTER

I remember Dr. R's words prior to going in. "The surgery will take a long time," he said. "And when it's over, you'll be on anti-rejection meds for the rest of your life."

He said it as a statement of fact. Not to scare me. Just so I couldn't say I didn't know.

"These medications are strong," he went on. "They work, but they also suppress your entire immune system. It's a trade-off. You get the new face—but your body's defenses go down. Way down."

I nodded, letting that sink in. I'd already lived through hell once. Wasn't planning on doing that again.

"The last thing we want," he said, "is for you to survive this surgery, only to die from something simple like a sinus infection or a stomach bug. Even a cold virus could be fatal without immunity."

"So, what happens?" I asked. "You put me in a bubble?"

He didn't smile. Just nodded.

"You'll be in a pressurized room with its' own air system and your own nurse. There will be a strict infection protocols so anyone who comes in will have to be cleared and approved in advance. No walk-ins. No surprises."

"Like the burn unit?" I asked.

"Similar, yes. Only more controlled. We'll need signed consent forms for any visitors. I want you to start making a list."

I thought about it. "There's Lori, of course, and Shannon. Bill. Travis. Jimmie…"

He scribbled the names down like he'd done this a thousand times.

"It's not just the surgery we're preparing you for, Pat," he said. "It's the life after. That's the part people don't always think through."

But not long before I would be wheeled back for surgery, Dr. R had shown up with news he needed to share before they began.

"Pat," he said, "I want to talk to you about the anti-rejection protocol again. We're going to do something different this time."

"Different good or different risky?"

He gave a small laugh. "Both."

I raised an eyebrow. He leaned forward, setting the clipboard he carried aside. "Most patients who've had this kind of surgery, we gave them a standard mix of steroids and something called antithymocyte globulin. It knocks out T cells—basically shuts down part of your immune system."

"Let me guess. Didn't work so great?" I asked.

"Not once. Every single patient had acute rejection, and fast."

I sat with that. All the science in the world, and still no guarantees.

"So what are we doing instead?"

"We're adding a drug called rituximab. It's usually used for high-risk kidney transplants. It doesn't just go after T cells—it targets B cells too."

"And that matters because…?"

"Because B cells can hide out in the skin. Sometimes they're the ones triggering rejection, and we don't catch it in time. Rituximab clears them out." He paused, then said, "There's little downside to trying it. One dose, the day after surgery. It might not stop rejection completely, but if we can buy you a year—or even just several good months—that's a win."

"You're just hoping it gives me more time?"

"Yes," he said. "That's the goal. We can't stop rejection from happening. But maybe we can push it far enough down the line that you get to live a real life before it shows up."

I let out a breath and nodded. "Then let's do it."

TWENTY-SIX HOURS after they wheeled me into that operating room, they wheeled me out to recovery and told my family and friends who were waiting that the surgery had gone well, better than expected. But there was still a long way to go. I was in the ICU, but this wasn't just any ICU. This was an extra special souped-up ICU. The nurses rotated shifts, but were basically the same three nurses on repeat, so we got to know each other really well. I felt like a VIP.

They kept me knocked out for a while to begin healing. They said my face was too swollen. They were right. Felt like it took up half the room. Skin pulled so tight, I thought it'd tear right down the middle. Couldn't move much. Couldn't talk. Didn't want to. They said it was normal. All part of it.

Shannon and Lori were the first to see me after the surgery. Told me how much they loved me. As they said their goodbyes, I lifted my hand and pounded my chest twice, right over my heart. I didn't have the words yet, but I hoped they got the message.

*I love you, too.*

"YOU'RE HEALING," Dr. Rodriguez told me.

I didn't feel like I was healing. I felt like I'd been hit by a bus and left out in the sun. But I reached for the dry-erase board I once again had lying next me, just like those days in the beginning when I couldn't talk, couldn't see, but could still scrawl out my thoughts with a marker. "Get me up." I had made the PT guy promise, and if Dr. R said I was healing, I wanted out of that bed.

ABOUT FOUR DAYS LATER, the doctors came in and started doing their rounds, checking if blood was still flowing to all parts of my face. Wondering if I could move various muscles yet. Dr. R took a risk.

"You can try to open your eyes if you want," he said. His voice was quiet. He didn't want to get either of our hopes too high, but he was eager to see what was possible. "Just try. No pressure."

So, I did.

Not sure how. Those were muscles I hadn't used in years, now under new skin, stitched up and swollen. But I kept pushing. And finally, something gave. Everything went bright. I blinked. Once. Then twice. The light was hitting hard, causing me to squint. My awe was overpowering the sting. For a second, I thought I was dreaming. The room didn't feel real.

I could see a blur in front of me move. Dr. R was observing my reaction. He didn't believe that I was able to blink so easily or quickly. Minimal movement was all he expected, but instead he witnessed full blinks.

My eyelids were his biggest gamble. Most face transplant patients don't get working eyelids. But he gave it everything—grafted muscle and skin, sewn with the precision of a watchmaker and the pressure of a world watching.

My eyes had survived the fire, but like the rest of me, they had come out with scars of their own. Burned, scarred, and dried out. Two weeks of damage inside a body that hadn't stopped burning once the fire was out. My left eye still carries a scar. But here's what I've learned—eyes are built to heal, if you give them the chance. The cornea's tough. It's a fighter.

I heard Jimmie. He had been in the room watching the doctors examine, poke and prod. "...Damn."

I turned my head, just enough to look at him.

He was staring at me like he'd seen a ghost. "Your eyes," he said, almost whispering. "Man, I forgot...I forgot they were that blue."

I didn't say anything. Couldn't, really. When I didn't have functioning eyelids, the opening for me to see out of had been small, not much larger than the end of a pencil eraser. Not big enough for anyone to see the bright blue of my irises for fourteen years.

"Would you like to see yourself?" Dr. Rodriquez asked. He handed me a mirror, and I slowly raised it in front of me.

Jimmie and Dr. R watched my every move. *My face.* I was still swollen and bruised around the eyes, but I could see... me. It was like seeing someone you recognize but can't quite place how you know them. It was familiar and strange all at once. I gently touched my cheek. Then, my forehead. My fingers slowly slid down the flesh of my nose. It felt different, almost as if touching a body part that's numb—like if your foot fell asleep. Although I barely felt it, I sure did see it. And it was mine.

The doctors explained that I would be a "blend" of what the donor looked like, and what my face had been. The new skin was laid over my bone structure, and much of what people look like comes from their underlying bones. That is how scientists can reconstruct what some ancient person might have looked like from their skull alone. I wouldn't look exactly like the old me , but I wouldn't look like David either. In fact, as the swelling continued to go down, I began to look like my younger boys. I was finally recognizable as a person again. But not just any person, I was once again... a Hardison.

My recovery continued, and one day looked like the next. Only the big moments stood out—some not because they were great, but because they were uncomfortable. Like all those damn swallow tests.

The feeding tube and IV drips were providing my nutrition and hydration, but they were beginning to do these swallow tests to see if I could drink something on my own. I had nightmarish flashbacks to that nasty gummy paste they made me swallow in The Med.

My mouth felt like it was stuffed with cotton. Not the soft kind—

the crunchy, dry kind you find out in the fields in Mississippi. I wanted water.

"I can't give you that, man," Jimmie said. He was sitting in the corner, legs kicked out, arms crossed like a bouncer.

"Sure you can," I told him.

"You know I can't."

"I'm asking."

"You can ask all day."

We went back and forth like that for a while. I could see him getting tense. He didn't want to be the one who had to hold the line. But I was mad. Dry. Miserable. And nobody was listening.

Finally, Jimmie stood up and walked out. Didn't say anything. I figured he was leaving to get a coffee or cool off.

He came back with a nurse.

She looked tired as if she was the one who had been having this argument with me for the last half hour.

"We've been through this," she said. "You haven't passed your swallow test yet. If we give you water, it might go down the wrong way and you could choke."

"I'll risk it," I said.

"Pat, that's not how this works."

"Still my body."

That got a long sigh.

Then Jimmie stepped in. Pulled her aside into the hallway.

I watched them through the glass. Couldn't hear, but I didn't have to. He was doing that thing he does—arms folded, head tilted, talking low and serious. She was shaking her head at first. Then slowly, she stopped.

They came back in. She held a cup. "You want it? Fine. But you only get a sip."

I nodded like a stubborn mule.

She held the straw up to my mouth.

I took a drink, but instantly regretted it. It hit the back of my throat and went sideways. I started coughing, hard. Tried to stop, but couldn't. Choked. Hacked. Spit water all over the front of my gown and down my chest. I started gasping. My eyes watered. It felt like I had swallowed fire. I grabbed at the bed rail, wheezing, trying to catch air.

Finally, I settled. Looked up at both of them. They didn't say a word—just stood there, arms crossed, waiting.

Jimmie raised an eyebrow. "Want any more?"

I glared at him. "Nope."

And I didn't ask again. Not till they said I could.

THE SWELLING CONTINUED to go down, but I had to relearn everything—how to smile, how to talk, how to move the muscles in my face. My nerves were attached to my muscles, and my muscles to my new face. It was a conscious effort to move my mouth, my nose, my cheeks, and my eyelids. But it worked. What had been another man's face was slowly and surely beginning to feel like mine.

They started me on the bike early—too early, if you ask them. The therapist left me alone for forty-five minutes, came back, and I'd already clocked five miles.

"Pat," he said, blinking at the screen, "you're supposed to ease into this."

"I ain't got time for 'ease'," I told him. "I've got kids."

He shook his head and walked off.

That was how most of rehab went. Some days I fought it. Some days I threw things. Some days I just stared out the window and didn't talk to anybody. I wasn't always nice. I wasn't always right. But I didn't quit. And I did something that seemed impossible. I passed the swallow test. It felt good to finally swallow that water without choking. Feeding tubes came out and I began to eat and drink like a fully functioning person. I started to feel normal again.

THEY SAID I was ahead of schedule. Said they'd never seen someone heal this fast. They said I'd be there six months. Maybe more. But I was doing in days what they thought would take weeks. Months of rehab done in half the time. But it didn't feel fast to me. It felt like a fight every single day. A fight to move. A fight to eat. A fight to feel like a human being again. But I kept showing up. Kept pushing. Not because I was strong—but because I had a reason. I wasn't doing this just to prove I could. I was doing it for the people waiting for me back home. For my kids. For the life I still wanted to live. I had made it through the fire. I had made it through the surgery. And now, I was fighting to come back. Not as the man I used to be. But as someone who could look his children in the eye again—and finally see the reflection of himself looking back.

## 27

# A DAD

"Later, I would like my kids to come. But not at first." I told Dr. R as we discussed my case in that conference room in Baltimore all those years before.

"No, I wouldn't advise them coming right away, but we will get them up there and help you prepare them for seeing your new face."

"How's the swelling?" Chrissi asked as we spoke on the phone about a month after the surgery.

"Going down, but look, I am still firm that it isn't time for the kids to come see me."

"Your surgery was over a month ago, Pat. They miss you."

"I know. I miss them, too, but I want to be able to walk and talk and not look like something out of a horror movie. You know how it was last time." The sound of Averi screaming at the sight of me rang in my ears. I couldn't put her through that again. Couldn't put any of them through that.

"I understand," she said.

"We will get them up here as soon as possible. It won't be much longer. Tell them I love them."

· · ·

It was October when I was finally ready for them to see my new face. Alison flew up with Lori and my mom. Chrissi brought our four kids up with her a few days later. She had shown them a picture the night before, so they would know what to expect.

I didn't sleep much.

That morning, I got up and got dressed. Paced around the room, trying to calm my nerves.

Then I heard the door click.

Cullen came in first.

He was the one I worried about the most. He had never seen me look any different than I had with the scars. He was still young enough for this to mess with his head. He stepped in and walked right up to me and gave me a hug.

"Hey bud," I said, my voice rough.

"Okay," he said, real quiet. "It's you."

That's all I needed. Didn't matter how I looked. Didn't matter what the world said. My kid knew me.

The others came in. Hugged me. Cried. They led Averi in with her eyes closed. She clung to me, listening to my voice first, so glad that I was okay. My face was the least of her concerns, but she wanted to connect to *me* first, then see my new face.

For the next few months, the kids flew up to see me while I was in rehab. Those visits meant everything. I still couldn't do much, but just seeing them—watching them light up when they saw me, hearing "Dad!"—told me I hadn't lost the thing that mattered most, my kids.

One weekend, the hospital pulled out all the stops. Shut down the whole street. Turned it into a block party for the staff and the fire department. There were food trucks, music, balloons—like a fair right in the middle of Manhattan.

The fire chief of the entire city came out to meet me. Said he'd heard about what happened and wanted to shake my hand. That alone would've been enough. But then he motioned toward one of the engines parked nearby. "We've got a seat saved for you," he said.

My kids piled in the back, grinning ear to ear. The sirens weren't for an emergency this time—they lit them up just for us. Rolled down the street, folks cheering from the sidewalks, the lights bouncing off the buildings like it was a parade. Later that day, they took the kids down to the harbor to tour the fireboat. The boat sprayed water halfway to the sky.

The chief invited me and Jimmie to tour the fire station. We visited with the guys and just talked shop. Then the tones dropped. Chief turned to me, "Want to go?"

"Are you kidding?" I felt like a kid again, with butterflies of nerves and excitement combined in my stomach. I climbed into the cabin and rode to the fire. I couldn't suit up, or fight alongside them, but they also didn't try to protect me, or coddle me, and I appreciated that.

That's the thing about firemen. Doesn't matter if you're from a small town in Mississippi or the biggest city in the country—when you're one of them, you're one of them. Brotherhood doesn't know state lines.

WE HAD dinners with Dr. Rodriguez and the team. One night, Jimmie and I got in an Uber on the way to meet them, and a yellow cab sideswiped us. Scraped the whole side of the car.

Jimmie just looked at me and shook his head. "Only us," he muttered.

That night, I gave Dr. R my old fire helmet. "For you," I said. "Hang it in your office."

"I will," he promised. I saw an interview he did a little while after that, and sure enough, in the background, hanging on the wall of his office, was my helmet.

. . .

THERE WERE SO many pieces to the puzzle of putting me back together, and as thorough as the team of doctors and specialists were, there were things we all missed. We were sitting there that night, planning on heading home, and Jimmie looked over at Dr. R and said, "Hey, how is he going to get through security? His ID doesn't match his face."

Dr. R and I both froze, staring at Jimmie.

Dr. R responded, "I hadn't thought about that. Let me make some phone calls and see if we can get it sorted out."

He got on the phone and got some senator involved. When we got to Newark to fly out, the head of the TSA met us at the gate and took us through a separate screening so they could check all my medications and everything. But I was allowed to fly home and deal with correcting my identification later.

It also helped that my story was becoming known as I went from one media event to another and my face, both the old one and the new one, was on every TV screen. But without getting that senator involved, who knows, I might have had to drive back to Mississippi.

WE GOT HOME the night before Thanksgiving. I wanted to fly in, hug my kids, and get home. No fanfare, no fuss.

But when I came down the escalator at the Memphis International Airport, I saw the crowd as I descended into baggage claim. Balloons, banners, welcome home signs, with my kids all standing in the front of the crowd. And everyone there was wearing these little plastic fire helmets. As they saw me coming, they began cheering.

Outside, they had a limo waiting. I was riding home in style.

When we pulled into town, it was like the Christmas parade. People were lined up on both sides of the road. Fire trucks. Lights. Banners. Kids waving little flags. I glared at Jimmie. He shrugged. "This was never up to you, Pat." *Guess not.* I blinked at the lights, waving at people who hadn't seen my real face in fifteen years.

. . .

AFTER I GOT HOME, I felt like a better dad. If you don't feel human, you don't show up as your best self. Small inconveniences annoy you and can cause you to lash out at those you love the most. Big ones can make you a terror. When you feel more like yourself, like the man God made you to be, then you show up differently—more calm, more confident, able to deal with the challenges of everyday life. It doesn't change your circumstances or the people around you, but it changes how you interact with them, and that means everything.

YOU MIGHT BE old enough to remember in the '80s when someone would win the Super Bowl and the reporter would say, "Dan, you just won the Super Bowl, what are you going to do now?" And he would respond, "I'm going to Disney World!" That is what we did. I had won the surgery lottery, and so, we went to Disney World. It was arranged by the people in New York. A trip for me and the kids to celebrate coming through the surgery. We hit all the parks and walked 'til our feet hurt. But it was something simple that I remember most... swimming.

There was a pool at the hotel, and of course the kids all wanted to get in. I hesitated at first. I hadn't been swimming in years. Couldn't go with the trach. But the trach was gone now, just a scar remained to show where it had once been.

"Come on, Dad. Get in," they begged.

I paused and stared at the water, which had seemed to be my kryptonite since the accident. Between not being able to swallow it or swim in it, it had been my arch-nemesis. There it was—the bright blue, glistening devil, taunting me. *Water can't put out my fire.* I cannonballed in. For the first time in fifteen years, I went swimming with my kids.

# 28

# A SPEAKER

"Of course, another reason for the security in the hospital during your recovery will be to shield you from the media," Dr. Rodriguez said, as he explained the balance between care and public attention.

"There was lots of media attention when I was injured, but it eventually died down—and Chrissi and my family handled most of those requests," I replied.

"They will be interested in this," he assured me. "Since this is research, everything will be documented. We'll control when the big moments go public."

THEY HELD off on press coverage until I had a few months of healing under my belt. When the time came, NYU Langone Public Relations team took the lead—scheduling press releases, interviews, media-ready photos, and video clips. My first public remarks were brief at a controlled press conference, then I was ushered behind the curtain while PR handled follow-up questions.

. . .

I WAS SITTING in the hotel room when my phone rang. It was a number I didn't recognize. Normally, I wouldn't have answered—too many calls were coming in from reporters, strangers, and media people trying to get a quote or a photo. But for some reason, I picked it up.

"Hello?"

A voice came on, smooth and confident. "Hi, is this Pat Hardison?"

"It is." I didn't say more than that. My voice must've told him I wasn't in the mood for games.

"This is Dr. Oz—from The Dr. Oz Show. I'm not sure if you've heard of it?"

I paused. "Uh, yeah. I've heard of it." But I still wasn't sure I believed it was him. What was Dr. Oz doing calling me personally? Where was his producer? His assistant? I waited, still suspicious.

"I've been following your case," he continued, friendly and polished. "It's remarkable. I'd love to have you come on the show. We think it could really inspire people."

That should've felt like a big moment. Like something worth celebrating. But I didn't feel anything except...uneasy.

I'd barely started to wrap my head around what had happened. The surgery. The healing. The stares. And now a national TV doctor wanted to put me in front of millions?

"I'll let the guys at NYU know about your request," I said. "All media has to go through them."

I don't think he expected that answer. I didn't care. I wasn't doing this for fame. I wasn't looking to be anyone's inspiration. I just wanted to be able to walk outside without scaring little kids.

I hung up the phone and called Dr. Rodriguez.

"Doc," I said, "you're not gonna believe this. Dr. Oz just called me himself."

He laughed. "You're getting popular, Pat."

"Y'all said to send everything through you," I reminded him. "So that's what I'm doing."

He thanked me, then told me they already had something in the works. "We're lining up an interview with a major network. Trust us—we'll handle it."

That was good enough for me. I didn't need to be famous. I just needed to breathe.

A FEW WEEKS LATER, entrenched in rehab, I was brought to a studio set within the hospital. Juju Chang of *Nightline* was conducting the interview. A full production team was there along with the whole works—cameras, lights, and microphones. NYU set up a room for us at the hospital. She sat across from me, warm and easy to talk to. Asked about the fire. The surgery. My kids.

It felt more like a conversation than an interview. Then slowly, the intensity of the questions increased. "Patrick, after fourteen years of living without a face, what was it like to finally look at yourself again?" she asked, her tone steady and gentle.

My answer came from a place deeper than words: "You get up every day of your life hating the way you look... and I'd do whatever it took to change that"— the raw truth I'd shared with *People* earlier.

As the interview wrapped, the crew pressed for emotional moments. "I still have the same friends. I still do the same things. I'm just Pat—and I'll always be Pat."

That segment ended up winning an Emmy for Outstanding Feature Story in a Newscast. Not because of me—but because they thought the story mattered. That's when I started to realize that maybe this whole ordeal was less about me and more about others.

NOT LONG AFTER THAT, we were staying at a hotel near the hospital when one of the guys glanced out the window and said, "There's paparazzi outside."

I laughed. "Must be someone famous here."

But when we stepped out the front doors, flashbulbs exploded in our faces. They were there for me.

My friends rushed to shield me, guiding me into the car as cameras clicked from every direction.

It felt unreal. I hadn't gone looking for fame. I just wanted to feel human again. But suddenly, I was living like a celebrity, and I didn't know how to handle it.

The transplant had made me look more like a man again—but now I was being seen everywhere, and not always in ways I could control.

The hall buzzed softly with conversation—donor families, transplant recipients, hospital staff. It was a reception arranged by LiveOnNY for the five recipients of David Rodebaugh's gifts of organ donation. His mother, Nancy, would be meeting the people who had received her son's heart, kidneys, liver, corneas, and of course, face. The other families waited downstairs. I stood upstairs, away from the rest of the crowd. I would be introduced separately. She entered the hall where the hosts introduced her to the recipients and their families.

Finally, they asked me if I was ready. I nodded. They asked her too. She nodded, tears already filling her eyes. As I walked down the stairs, I saw her at the bottom, waiting anxiously. I couldn't imagine what she must be thinking.

Recognition and warmth unfolded across her face. She reached out, "Pat," she breathed, stepping forward to hug me. Her arms were firm, motherly.

She pulled back, eyes steady on mine. "Can I kiss your forehead?" she asked.

I nodded. She had said she would kiss David's forehead each night before she tucked him in. We also had the same scar on our foreheads. As a parent, I understood. How could I deny a mother that one gift in return for all she gave me?

. . .

BACK IN MISSISSIPPI, I realized I'd become somewhat of a local celebrity. Churches, Rotary clubs, veterans' groups, and even hospitals invited me to speak. Unexpectedly, I saw more of how much my story affected people—not because it was heroic, but maybe because it was raw.

Sometimes I spoke. At a major church in Jackson, I stood before a crowd and said, "I'm the same person I've always been... this was the outcome of doing what I loved."

But more often, I said no. Detailing the darkness—the addiction, the arrests, the failures—felt like ripping open old wounds. Yet, I knew they were part of the story—a necessary prelude to the transformation that allowed me to endure the transplant and its aftermath.

I wasn't a speaker. Didn't want to be. But here were people who needed to hear that life doesn't always end when you think it does—people who needed to hear that there is always hope to be found.

# PART VII
# THE COST OF SURVIVING

## 29

## THE FACE COLLAPSES

Dr. Rodriguez sat across from me, elbows resting on the edge of the desk. "Pat, I need to talk to you about something you probably already know is coming."

I nodded. "The pain meds."

He gave a small nod. "Yeah. This surgery's going to be intense. Long recovery. And you're going to need medication to manage that. Typically, strong meds are prescribed for something like this. Opioids."

I didn't say anything. Just stared at a spot on the floor between us.

"We've reviewed your history," he said gently. "We know the battles you've fought."

I looked up. "So, what—you think I'll relapse?"

"I think you've worked too hard to go back," he said. "Which is why we're putting some safeguards in place. Psychological evaluations. Structured dosing. A monitored support system. No wiggle room."

"No more taking the pills like I want," I muttered.

"No more calling the shots," he agreed. "You won't be in control of your medication. We will. That's not punishment, Pat—it's protection."

I took a breath and let it out slowly. "You think I can do this? With all that in place?"

"I wouldn't be here if I didn't," he said. "But I also know this part's going to be just as hard—maybe harder—than the surgery itself."

He let that settle.

I nodded again. "Okay. Just...don't let me go back there."

He extended his hand to shake on it. I grabbed his hand and looked into his eyes. "I don't plan to," he said.

By the next year, I felt it slipping again. Just like before. That quiet pull. That slow slide. Reaching for the pill bottle out of habit instead of necessity. I picked up the phone and called Dr. R. When he answered, I didn't waste time. "You gotta help me get off this mess," I said. "I'm going under again."

There was a pause on the other end. Then his voice came through, steady and calm. "Okay, Pat. Thank you for calling. That was the right thing to do."

For once, I'd told the truth. No half-answers. No pretending I had it under control.

My family didn't yell. Didn't scold. They just got me back into the hospital. Quietly. Safely.

No jail cell this time. No handcuffs. No guards pounding on bars. No seizures in the middle of the night.

Just support. Structure. Surrender.

They walked me through detox the right way. Surrounded me with people who knew the signs. Who didn't let me hide. Who didn't let me lie to myself.

And I stayed. Because I wanted to.

Because I was finally ready to stop falling.

That decision saved my life.

After the transplant, the first miracle came not from my face—but from my eyes. I flew up to Boston Sight, and they fitted me with special contacts—saline-filled lenses that helped protect and hydrate my eyes. When I first put them in, I felt instant cooling relief. I hadn't realized how much my eyes hurt until then.

Before the transplant, contacts were never an option because the holes around my eyes were too small. Now, I realized my eyes had been burning from the dryness for years.

My vision slowly came back. First shapes. Then details. Eventually, I hit 20/30. Better than it had been in years.

It is not perfect. Mornings are still the worst. I wake up feeling like someone stuffed sand under my eyelids. Burning. Scratching. But once I get those lenses in, the fog lifts and faces come into focus.

BEFORE THE SURGERY, Dr. Rodriguez didn't sugarcoat anything.

"It's not if—it's when," he told me. "Your body doesn't forget. Eventually, it'll try to fight this."

He said I'd have five, maybe seven good years before rejection started. After that, I'd need more treatments. More meds. More appointments. Maybe more surgeries. At the time, I nodded. Took it in. But I didn't really let it settle. I was too focused on surviving.

I didn't have space to carry that weight too.

But then year five came. Year six. Then seven. Still nothing.

My doctors were amazed. They said I was breaking records. Said my tissue looked strong. Said I might be one of the lucky ones.

And I started to believe it.

I GOT USED to waking up and seeing a face in the mirror that felt like me. I started going out more. Talking more. Traveling. Speaking. I didn't think about the "when" anymore.

Until it showed up.

IT STARTED SLOWLY. My ears didn't quite sit the same. The shape softened. The edges blurred. Then my nose started to swell—just a little at first, then more. I knew it wasn't normal. I knew what it meant.

But I didn't say anything.

Started wearing my baseball cap a little lower. Kept my sunglasses on a little longer. I've always worn them, so nobody thought much of it. I played it off as just me being me.

But the truth was, I was hiding.

It's easy to keep secrets when folks are used to you not complaining.

Even now, I don't make a big deal about it. But I feel it. My face feels different. Tender in spots. Puffy and swollen again. It feels like it did right after the transplant, when everything was still raw.

Except this time, it's not settling in; it's coming undone. It's rejecting, just like Dr. R said it would.

## 30

## THE RUPTURE

In July of 2023—over two decades after the fire that started this whole story—I was sitting in my recliner, watching TV, waiting for Braden to get home from his shift at the steakhouse. I had no idea I was about to face another life-or-death struggle.

He came in around 11:30 p.m., tired, and stretched out on the couch in the living room. I stayed in my recliner so we could talk. Somewhere in the middle of the conversation, we both drifted off to sleep.

Around 1:30 a.m., I woke up to a strange warmth spreading across my T-shirt. I looked down and saw it was soaked in blood. My hand went to my neck, and I could feel it—blood spewing like water from a hose. Later, the doctors would explain that when the transplant tissue began to reject, the seam they'd sewn together had started to separate, opening blood vessels. One of them had ruptured.

I tried to wake Braden, but he was sleeping hard. I kept calling his name until he startled awake, jumping to his feet as his eyes took in the scene—blood everywhere. My living room looked like a murder scene from TV.

Braden called 911. We both thought this might be it. I couldn't stop the bleeding. The dispatcher toned out the fire department and the ambulance. The fire crew arrived first. Howard Boling came in and sat me down; I was lightheaded and dizzy by then. He held pressure on my neck for what felt like forever—13 to 15 minutes—until the ambulance pulled up. The bleeding had slowed but hadn't stopped.

While we waited, I kept trying to call Chrissi. I wanted to say a few things in case I didn't make it. Her ringer was off, so I called her mom. When I finally got Chrissi on the phone and let her know what was happening, she and her mom jumped in the car and headed our way. There was so much I wanted to tell her—that I hated how things had ended, that I hated losing my family and being divorced, and that if I could do anything to fix it, I would. But some things just can't be fixed, and we have to learn to live without the ones we love.

They loaded me into the ambulance and were pulling away as Chrissi and her mom were pulling into the driveway. They stayed behind to help clean the mess before coming to the hospital.

I'd lost a lot of blood by the time the doctors got me stable. The ruptured artery fed part of the graft—right in the transplanted tissue. The doctors told me if it had gone on much longer, I might not have made it. They cauterized the wound and sent me home.

BUT NOT TOO LONG after that; it opened again. This time, they sent me to The Med, back to the place where this all began. I had to have emergency surgery. A new skin graft to patch what the bleeding tore up. They kept me for a few days, watching for signs of deeper rejection, running labs, monitoring the pressure behind the skin.

When they released me, I left with more meds, a swollen face, and a fresh warning: "We're entering a new phase."

They were right.

Back at home, I took the prescription for those pain pills and handed it off to Chrissi.

Even though we weren't together anymore, she was still someone I could trust when it counted. "Keep these. Don't give me one unless I call and ask—and even then, make sure I mean it," I instructed.

She nodded and smiled.

That was a big moment for me. Because though the pain was real, the fear was worse. I remembered where those pills took me last time—and I wasn't about to go back there. Not for anything.

Recovery was slow.

I STAYED HOME, face wrapped, swollen, sore down to the bone. Not much to do but rest, drink water, and wait. The skin graft held, thank God. But my doctors made it clear—we were on borrowed time now. The signs of rejection were no longer just possible. They were here and they were unrelenting. That initial rupture had been just the first crack in the dam.

The doctors never promised forever. Back when I signed the papers for the transplant, they told me straight: "We're hoping for five to seven good years. Ten if we are lucky."

I had been okay with that.

But then nine years came and went.

A week and a half later, my artery explodes.

That's not nothing.

CHRISSI and I sat all the kids down. We didn't sugarcoat it. Didn't give 'em speeches or hold hands in a circle. We just sat at the kitchen table and told them the truth.

"This thing might not last forever," I said. "Could be another year. Could be ten more. We don't know."

They didn't say much at first.

After a while, one kid asked if I was scared.

I said, "I ain't scared of dying."

They nodded, like they expected that.

Then I added, "But I'll tell you what I *am* scared of—being locked up in my own house, too sick to live and too stubborn to die. That's worse than anything."

They got quiet again.

I think that was the moment reality hit them. That we've already had more time than most people thought we would.

WITHIN A FEW WEEKS, the phone rang. New York wanted me back up there. Said we needed to begin anti-rejection treatments—stronger steroids, more immune suppression, injections, infusions.

Ten years ago, everything was urgent. A fight for survival. The surgery, the rehab, the press, the questions. Everything was loud. Everything moved fast. But this time?

Now it was quiet.

They flew me in; put me in a little apartment tucked behind the hospital. White walls. Cold floors. A stiff bed. I stayed for about a month. On most of those days, I didn't leave the apartment unless it was for treatment. Those consisted of an IV and time in a chair waiting for it to run, almost like chemo. They hooked me up, and fluids would run in. The steroids would hit me hard—make me shaky, flushed, short of breath. They'd run labs and check pressures and ask how I was sleeping.

Sometimes we go out to eat with people I had met on the journey —JuJu Chang, Dr. R, the trustees of the myFace organization.

Sometimes I would still give interviews. Once, Sean Hannity came in with his team for an interview. We joked and laughed as if we had been friends for years.

Mostly, I sat in the quiet of the apartment alone, wishing I was home with my kids.

The hardest part was the waiting. Between appointments, there wasn't not much to do but sit with it. Sit with the fear. The not knowing. The face I fought so hard to keep finally started to let go.

I could look in the mirror and see the difference. The nose hadn't held its shape. I had lost part of my ears. My face was swollen again. The swelling changed the way my eyes looked—made me look tired all the time. Hiding behind my baseball cap and sunglasses again was not to fool anybody. It was just to feel a little more in control.

. . .

It wasn't a one-time trip either. It was regularly—every few months. I didn't tell many people what those trips were like. Not because I was ashamed but because it was hard to explain what it felt like to be both a miracle and a man falling apart at the same time.

They told me once that this face could give me five good years. It stretched to nine before the rejection started. I'm proud of that. But now I'm back in another fight—and once again I don't know what the outcome may be. This time's not about cameras and headlines like the surgery had been. This time, it's about holding on.

## 31

## PAT

Mornings are my favorite. I get up early, same as I always have. Doesn't matter if I've got somewhere to be or not. I like the quiet. I like the stillness before the world starts moving. I make a pot of coffee and step out onto the porch of my little apartment. It's nothing fancy. Just a small place I built on my land. One bedroom. A little living room and kitchen. It's enough.

I sit out there most mornings, cup in hand, steam rising, watching the sun climb up over the trees. Sometimes I hear the birds. Sometimes it's just the wind rustling through the leaves. Those are the moments I feel most like myself. Not the old me. Not the one before the fire. Just...me. The true core of who God made...and remade.

I DON'T HAVE kids anymore.

I mean, I do—but they're all grown up now. My youngest is old enough to order a beer with dinner. They've got jobs, bills, marriages. They're out living their lives—the way I hoped they would.

But the real prize? The grandbabies.

The first time I held my oldest grandbaby, it was like holding her mama all over again—those perfect blue eyes, the wisps of blonde hair. She looked up at me like I was the safest place on earth. Tiny hand wrapped around my finger. No fear. Just love.

They say grandkids are the reward for raising your own kids. Some folks even say they're better than having kids—and let me tell you something: they're right.

Each of my three oldest kids now has a kid of their own. That's three little lights in my life that I never could've imagined during the hard years. They don't know the old me. They don't remember the accident or the surgeries. They didn't have to live through the turmoil my kids did. They don't know what I looked like before—or after. All they know is Papa. The one who shows up with toys at Christmas, who sneaks them candy from his pocket when Mama's not looking, who sits them up on his lap and lets them drive the lawnmower—even if it's not turned on.

There's nothing in the world like it.

Now I get to be the one that shows up—that is there when my kids call and need someone to help out. The one who watches the grandkids during the day if their parent needs to run errands, or picks them up from school, or just be the one they come sit with when they're tired and need a snack and a cartoon. I've learned the names of their favorite shows. I've got juice boxes in the fridge. And I've got the kind of patience I didn't have when I was young and life was spinning fast.

There's just something different about being Papa. You're not trying to shape them or teach them every life lesson. You're just loving them. Being present. Making memories they'll carry long after I'm gone.

WHEN I'M NOT HELPING with the grandkids, I help my son detail cars —got his own thing going to make a little cash before he heads off for new adventures. I can't do some of the heavy scrubbing, but I can still wash a windshield, spray down the mats, and make things look sharp. I still know how to sell. So, I do what I can to spread the word and tell folks around town where to go if they want their car done right.

It's not the kind of retirement some people dream about with beach houses, golf carts and timeshares. But I'm not most people. I've already had a second chance at life and I know nothing matters more than being with these kids of mine.

FRIDAY NIGHTS, you'll usually find me at Como Steakhouse.

It's just down Highway 51 from Senatobia, tucked in the middle of that old downtown strip. Folks around here know it well. I think just about everybody in my family's worked there at one point or another. Hostess, server, busboy, line cook—you name it, one of my kids has done it. Some of them still do.

By the time I pull into the parking lot, they've already got the big round table in the back saved for us. They know we're coming. There's never fewer than eight or ten of us. Sometimes more. Friends, family, girlfriends, boyfriends, and kids' friends who might as well be family—we take up a good bit of space.

There's something about sitting at that table, all packed in together, passing down foil-wrapped baked potatoes still steaming through the heat, splitting baskets of butter-soaked Texas toast, everyone fighting over whose steak tastes the best. I order the ribeye, same as I have for years. Medium. Load the potato up—cheese, sour cream, bacon, all of it. No sense in holding back when you've made it through what I have.

Everybody in that restaurant seems to know me. Or if they don't, they know somebody at the table. They stop by on their way to a booth or waiting on a to-go order. Shake my hand. Thump me on the back. Ask how the grandkids are doing. They don't ask how I'm doing physically anymore, and I can't tell you how much I appreciate that is no longer the main topic of conversation.

There was a time that was all people talked about. The surgeries, the meds, the transplant. Questions I didn't always have answers for. Now? It's just "How's your boy doing with the business?" or "Your granddaughter in preschool yet?" Regular stuff. Like I'm just Pat again. Not the guy with the burns, or the new face. Just...me.

Nobody stares in there. Nobody leans in and whispers. They've heard the story. Lived it with me, in a way. They know the whole deal—what I went through, what I came back from. And they also know we're all here to eat a good steak, laugh a little, and be with our people.

That round table in the back—that's one of my favorite places on earth. I sit there a few minutes after everyone else has left, just soaking in the hum of the place. Forks clinking, chairs scooting, folks heading out full and happy. I think about how many nights I've spent here over the years. How many more I might get. And I pray a simple prayer: Lord, keep pulling me out of the fire.

# EPILOGUE

I get messages sometimes. Emails, Facebook comments. They say things like, *"I thought I had a big problem, but after reading about you, I don't even want to complain anymore."* Or, *"You're such a hero. I could never be that brave."* I never know quite what to say back. Because I'm not a hero. I'm just a guy who falls asleep in the recliner with cartoons still playing on the TV.

I'm just Pat.

Yeah, I had an accident. A bad one. It changed my life in ways I'll never fully explain. It led to a groundbreaking surgery that drew attention from around the world. But I was doing what I loved. I was trying to help somebody. And if I could go back, I'd still run into that burning house. Every time.

THAT DOESN'T MEAN I wasn't angry. I was angry for years. Angry at what I lost. At the pain. At how hard everything became. The pain still gets me sometimes, but now that pain is more about everything the accident cost me than anything physical. And when I am wallowing in that pain, God will humble me quick. Show me someone else that has it worse and remind me of all I still have. I know what it means to be spared when you shouldn't be. Makes you appreciate things more—the sunrise, your grandkid's giggle, working with your son, and even just getting up without hurting too bad. There have certainly been times I asked God, "*Why?*" But maybe that is the wrong question. Maybe the right question is, "*How?*" How will He use this unimaginable thing that happened to me?

I should've died in that fire. I should've died a dozen times since. But I didn't. And I don't think that's an accident.

God kept me here for a reason.

Not so I could be famous. Not so I could be on the news or write this book. Not even to have a surgery that advanced medical science. But so I could sit across from someone who's going through hell and tell them, "Don't give up. You're not alone." So I could show folks, that even after the worst thing you can imagine—there's still life. There's still love. There's still joy to be had.

Now, I stand and look in the mirror, and the glass isn't foggy or shattered. I certainly don't see the man I was before. But I don't see the man I was during the hard years, either. I can look at myself now, and what I see is a man who has fought fires—literally and figuratively. A man that has come out the other side, battered and scarred, and still fighting. But my hope? Is it to be remembered as a man that was a fighter? No. It's to be a man who can help those who are also *facing the fire.*

# PHOTOS

Many readers will look for the "before and after." Out of respect for the medical team and to keep those images in their proper context, we've chosen not to reprint clinical photographs here. To view NYU Langone Health's official pre- and postoperative images and timeline, please visit their website: https://nyulangone.org/news/one-year-later-heroic-firefighter-who-underwent-most-extensive-face-transplant-thriving or scan the QR code provided.

Included here are two of Pat's personal favorites:

- **Dress Whites**: Pat Hardison in his Senatobia Fire Department dress uniform. Used with permission of the Hardison family.
- **Papa**: Pat "Papa" Hardison with two of his grandkids. © Brandee Lott Photograph

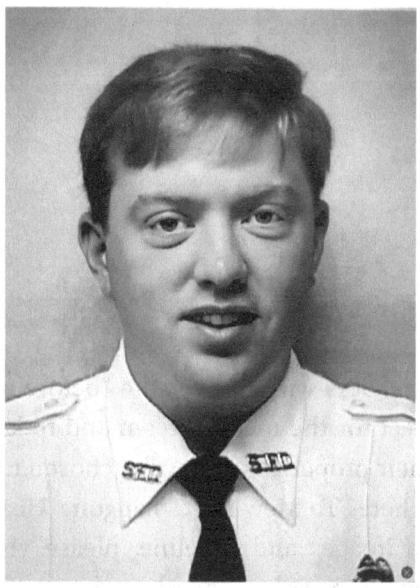

*Pat in dress whites, Senatobia Fire Department (1999). Photo courtesy of the Hardison family.*

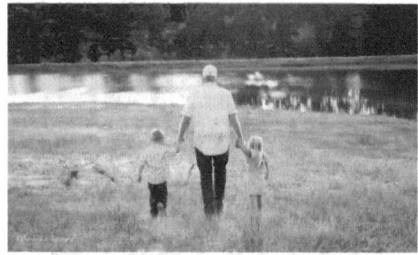

*"Papa" with two grandchildren (2025). Photo © Brandee Lott Photography. Used with permission*

# TIMELINE OF EVENTS

To clarify the order of events, here is a simple timeline for reference.

**1974**
Pat Hardison was born in Mississippi.

**1994**
Pat turned 20.
Bought his first home.
Daughter Alison was born.

1997
>  Son Dalton was born.

1998
>  Pat married Chrissi.

1999
>  Daughter Averi was born.

SEPTEMBER 5, 2001
>  Pat was severely burned while responding to a house fire.
>  9/11 occurred six days after the fire.
>  Hospitalized 63 days in the burn unit.
>  Returned home in time for Thanksgiving and Christmas.

2002
>  Began wearing a pressure mask daily.
>  Learned to drive again—first outing was a drive-thru.

2003
>  Son Braden was born.
>  Pat started a new shop.

2004
>  Sold the Yellow Dog house and moved in with Chrissi's parents.
>  Son Cullen was born.

2005–2006

Built a new house in the Bartlett Woods subdivision.

The housing market later collapsed; the house was lost to foreclosure.

**2006**

Pat moved in with his parents; Chrissi and the kids moved in with hers.

**2008**

Pat checked into rehab but left early—on his and Chrissi's tenth anniversary.

Divorce finalized.

**2011**

Pat's father passed away—on his mother's birthday.

**2012**

Family friend Clay Moore contacted Dr. Eduardo Rodriguez (NYU).

Dr. Rodriguez reached out to begin evaluation.

**2014**

Approved for a full face transplant at NYU Langone.

Placed on the transplant waitlist with LiveOnNY.

**AUGUST 14–15, 2015**

Underwent a 26-hour face transplant at NYU Langone.

Returned home to Mississippi the day before Thanksgiving, 2015.

. . .

**2023**

Experienced signs of rejection.

Suffered a ruptured artery; resumed regular treatments in New York.

**July 2024**

Pat's mother passed away, shortly before he began this book.

# ACKNOWLEDGMENTS

First off, I want to thank God. I should've been dead, but He had other plans. I've been through hell and back, and I never walked it alone. I've seen too much to believe any of this happened by chance.

To Mom, Dad, Lori, and Shannon—thank you for loving me when I wasn't easy to love. You carried me more times than I can count.

To Chrissi—thank you for walking through the fire with me. We didn't make it through as husband and wife, but you stood by me in the hardest years of my life. I'll always be grateful.

To my kids—Alison, Dalton, Averi, Braden, and Cullen—you're the reason I kept going. I know it wasn't easy. I missed things I can't get back. I love you with everything I've got.

To my grandkids—you bring light into my life. You're pure joy. You remind me why second chances matter.

To my friends who never quit on me—Bill Weeks, Jimmie Neal, and Travis McDonald, and many others not specifically mentioned in the book—thank you for showing up, again and again.

To Ronnie Warren—thank you for opening the door and giving me my start in the fire service.

To the men and women of the Senatobia Fire Department—my SFD family—thank you for the way you prayed for me, checked on me, and kept me part of the crew. You know who you are.

To Clay Moore—thank you for making that call and getting the ball rolling. You helped open a door I couldn't open on my own.

To my UT doctors in Memphis—Dr. William Wallace, Dr. James Fleming, and Dr. Bill Hickerson and his team—thank you for the steady care and skill. You kept me going when the road was long.

To my NYU team—Dr. Eduardo Rodriguez, Dr. Bruce Gelb, and the entire transplant team at NYU Langone—you gave me more than a face. You gave me a second shot at life. I'll never forget what you did for me.

A special thanks to the folks who sat for interviews and helped us get the story right: Jimmie Neal; Bill Weeks and his wife; Clay Moore; Chief Copeland and Neal; Matt Hale—thanks for clearing up what happened inside the house that day; Chrissi—thank you for hours on the phone, telling the hard parts; Lori—thank you for showing up, reading drafts, and helping us get it right; Travis McDonald; and Ronnie Warren. Your memories and honesty mattered.

To our editor, Gregory Gobin—your notes turned a so-so draft into a story our beta readers couldn't put down.
  To our cover designer, Kevin Pitts—your cover idea nailed it.
  To Brandee Lott—thanks for jumping in on a moment's notice and getting the shots we needed.
  To our amazing beta readers—your feedback made this book stronger.

To my friends and family back home—thank you for your prayers, your support, and your stubborn belief that I'd make it. Every church around prayed for me. I wish I could list every name. Please know I felt it. None of this would've been possible without you.

And to Carolyn Wiley—and her husband, Bryan—thank you for helping me tell my story and for pushing this book across the finish line. You kept my voice in it when I didn't have the words. I couldn't have done this without you.

If I missed your name, I'm sorry. I've had more help than I can count. Thank you, all of you, from the bottom of my heart.

—Pat

# ABOUT THE AUTHOR

Pat Hardison is a former volunteer firefighter from Senatobia, Mississippi, and the first person in the world to survive a full face transplant. After a fire in 2001 left him with severe burns and permanent disfigurement, Pat endured over 70 surgeries and became a pioneer in one of the most complex medical procedures ever attempted.

But Pat's story isn't just about what happened in the operating room—it's about what it took to keep going. Through years of pain, addiction, loss, and grace, Pat discovered that survival is more than staying alive. It's choosing to fight for something more.

Pat now shares his story of faith, resilience, and redemption to encourage others who are walking through fires of their own. He's a proud father of five, Papa to his grandkids, and a grateful man who knows that if you're still breathing, God's not finished.

instagram.com/hardison_pb
facebook.com/pat.hardison.9
tiktok.com/@patrickhardison47

# PUBLISHER'S NOTE

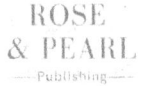

*Thank you for reading Pat's story.*

This book was created from many hours of conversations, interviews, and careful review. It is told in Pat's voice, as he lived it. Some names and small details have been changed or modified to protect privacy.

Pat never asked to be the center of attention. He's a dad and a firefighter at heart. What you've just read is not a medical case study or a headline—it's a man telling the truth about pain, grit, faith, and the people who helped him stand up again.

We honor the donor and his family, whose courage made Pat's transplant possible. We also honor the medical team who carried this work with skill and humility, and the firefighters, friends, and family who showed up when it counted.

If this book moved you, consider two simple next steps. First, talk with your family about organ donation and register in your state. Second, show up for someone who's hurting. A meal. A ride. A prayer. Small things change lives.

For speaking inquiries, bulk orders, or permissions, contact:
Rose & Pearl Publishing
support@roseandpearl.net
https://roseandpearlpublishing.com

With gratitude,

Carolyn Wiley, Ed.D.
Founder/CEO, Rose & Pearl Publishing
Mississippi

- instagram.com/roseandpearlpublishing
- facebook.com/carolynwileywrites
- tiktok.com/@carolyn_wiley
- youtube.com/@thepublishedpearl

www.ingramcontent.com/pod-product-compliance
Lightning Source LLC
Chambersburg PA
CBHW010243010526
44107CB00034B/1415/J